Psychology as Applied to Nursing

Andrew McGhie MA, PhD
Professor of Psychology, Queen's University, Kingston, Ontario;
Formerly Director of the Department of Clinical Psychology,
Royal Dundee Liff Hospital

Psychology as Applied to Nursing

Andrew McGhie

Seventh Edition

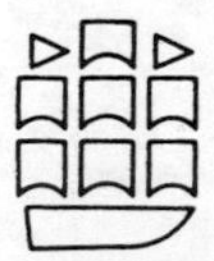

CHURCHILL LIVINGSTONE
EDINBURGH LONDON AND NEW YORK 1979

CHURCHILL LIVINGSTONE
Medical Division of Longman Group Limited

Distributed in the United States of America by
Churchill Livingstone Inc., 19 West 44th Street,
New York, N.Y. 10036, and by associated
companies, branches and representatives
throughout the world.

First Edition 1959
Second Edition 1961
Third Edition 1963
Fourth Edition 1966
Fifth Edition 1969
Sixth Edition 1973
Seventh Edition 1979
Reprinted 1980

ISBN 0 443 01827 8

British Library Cataloguing in Publication Data

McGhie, Andrew
Psychology as applied to nursing. — 7th ed.
1. Nursing — Psychological aspects
I. Title
150'.2'4613 RT86 78—40418

Printed in Singapore by
Kyodo-Shing Loong Printing Industries Pte Ltd

Preface to the Seventh Edition

For this latest edition of the text, much of the material has been revised and updated. However, probably the most notable changes are in the form of two additional sections. One of these concerns the difficult questions which arise in dealing with the terminally ill patient. This has been added to the section on Communication in Chapter 12. Another major addition is in the chapter on Learning (Ch. 10), where an added section deals with nursing involvement in behaviour modification programmes.

In the recent British Psychological Society survey of nursing education in psychology, these were the main topics which nurses felt were neglected in their psychology texts. It was heartening to the author to observe that the same survey indicated that this book is still viewed favourably by nurses in training. Accordingly, I should like to close this short preface to the seventh edition by seriously thanking the many nursing readers whose interest has made each succeeding edition possible.

Kingston, Ontario A. McGhie
1978

Preface to the Seventh Edition

For this latest edition of the text, much of the material has been revised and updated. However, probably the most notable changes are in the form of two additional sections. One of these concerns the ethical questions which arise in dealing with the terminally ill patient. This has been added to the section on communication in Chapter 12. Another major addition is in the chapter on Learning (Ch. 10), where an added section deals with nursing involvement in behaviour modification programmes.

In the recent British Psychological Society survey of nursing education in psychology, these were the main topics which nurses felt were neglected in their psychology teaching. It was heartening to the author to observe that the same survey indicated that this book is still widely used by nurses in Britain. Accordingly, I should like to close this short preface to the seventh edition by sincerely thanking the many nursing readers whose interest has made each succeeding edition possible.

Kingston, Ontario A. McGhie
1979

Preface to the First Edition

In the current syllabus of subjects for the preliminary examination for the Certificate of General Nursing there is a new additional subject entitled 'Psychology Applied to Nursing'. The already harassed student nurse who faces a formidable list of subjects will most likely welcome this new addition with all the enthusiasm and ardour usually reserved for matron's ward round. One can imagine the trainee nurse protesting 'I came here to learn to care for sick people, not to learn psychology!' What, then, is the justification for adding this subject to the nurse's training programme? This question is perhaps partly answered in the General Nursing Council's guide to the training syllabus from which the following statement is taken: 'This subject introduces the student nurse to the study of the individual as a person with a mind to be cared for as well as a body. . . . The aim is to help her (the nurse) to be more effective both in the nursing care that she gives to her patients and in dealing with her own day-to-day problems.' Put more briefly, it is hoped that some knowledge of psychology will increase the nurse's understanding of herself and others. This book is, then, principally directed at the student nurse as a contribution towards making the introduction of psychology in her training as painless as possible. As an author always hopes to sell his book in the widest market possible, let me hasten to add that it is hoped that qualified senior nurses and, dare we say it, nursing tutors might also find the material relevant and useful. Indeed, parts of the book are specifically designed to deal with the problems arising in supervisory nursing. As the author is a clinical psychologist working in a mental hospital, it is also hoped that the subject matter outlined will prove applicable to the revised training course for the Certificate of Mental Nursing which now gives much wider scope to psychological matters.

The next logical step would appear to be to define psychology as a subject, as there is often a great deal of confusion in people's minds regarding the differences between psychology, psychiatry and psycho-analysis. Psychiatry is essentially the study of the causes and treatment of mental illness. Psycho-analysis is a specific method of treating some forms of mental disturbance by helping the patient to recognise and overcome the unconscious mental forces which produce his symptoms. While these two subjects are concerned with abnormal mental processes, psychology is interested in normal mental processes and in the relationship between normal and abnormal behaviour. It studies mental disturbance only in relation to the larger background of normal human development. We might define psychology as 'the scientific study of human experience and behaviour'.

When one is asked one's occupation and replies that one is a psychologist the most frequent response is 'Oh, I'm a bit of a psychologist myself!' Although this is a little chastening to one's pride there is, of course, a large element of truth in the comment. We all study human experience and behaviour in our everyday life and frequently make assessments regarding the psychological attributes of others. This is particularly the case if our work is such as to bring us into continual contact with other people. Thus, the shopkeeper, the door-to-door salesman, the teacher, the nurse, and others are all in a sense using psychology in their work. This has caused some people to redefine psychology cynically as 'common sense messed around a bit'. The professional psychologist attempts to justify his existence by also observing and assessing human nature, but in as objective and scientific a way as possible. Many of our everyday observations and the opinions derived from them are distorted in the act of being made by our individual subjective bias, prejudices, and other 'blind spots'. We reach conclusions about people on scanty evidence, generalise these conclusions and neglect to test their validity. The psychologist may start with an opinion which is similarly formed and open to the same criticisms but he does not form conclusions until he has put his hypothesis (his 'hunch') to an objective and scientific test of verification. We have not the space here to go into any of the rather complicated experimental techniques which are used to test the validity of psychological theories. Most of them are based on statistical procedures which have made psychology increasingly a mathematical science. It is sufficient for our present purposes to make the point that psychological theory is not merely the result of woolly, armchair philosophising. Any conclusions reached are usually thoroughly sifted through the machinery of scientific verification before they are accepted. Psychology is, however, concerned with human behaviour and this is a commodity which is not always amenable to precise measurement and mathematical calculation. As a result of this a number of psychological conclusions do reach the other side of the sifting process with their inaccuracies and blemishes still intact. Curiously enough, it is often the wildest and least checked psychological ideas which are accepted by workers in other fields and become part of our folklore of unverified assumptions about human behaviour. In the chapters which follow we will try to dispose of some of these wild and often dangerous conceptions and help the reader to see the present state of psychological knowledge in a more balanced and limited perspective. Some degree of unverifiable opinion is, of course, inevitable in any subject which sets out to study such an unwieldy and unpredictable phenomenon as human behaviour. The present author has taken the same liberty in stating at times his own opinion on aspects of mental activity which cannot be directly observed.

The presentation of the material is in four main sections. The first, longest, and perhaps most important, section deals with psychological aspects of human development from the first months of life through the subsequent stages of childhood, adolescence, adulthood and old age. The second section deals with human motivation and considers some of the factors which move us to act in our individual ways. The last chapter of this section is concerned with the complementary functions of heredity and environment in moulding our personality, and this leads us on to consider in Part III some of the processes by which we become aware of, and deal with, our environment. In the final section we take a brief look at group processes, to remind us that we live not in a vacuum but as part of a complicated social pattern.

Psychological material presented to nurses is, in my experience, either coldly academic and difficult or so simplified as to resemble a tiny tots' comic paper. Over-simplification tends to produce more than one resemblance to a child's comic paper, for the simplicity is usually achieved at the expense of accuracy and the nurse must react with healthy laughter and scepticism to some of the information she is given under the name of psychology. My aim here has been to find a compromise in a presentation which is neither over-theoretical and abstruse nor over-simplified and inaccurate. Such a happy medium is difficult to find and the reader must be left to pronounce the final judgment. Technical jargon has been avoided as much as possible, but as some of the terms used may be unfamiliar to the reader a glossary is provided at the back of the book.

At the end of each chapter a few questions are presented to allow the reader the opportunity of formulating her opinions on the subject matter she has been reading. These questions might also be useful in giving the reader some experience with the type of questions which might well be asked in psychology examinations.

There remains but one comment which I must make to avoid the wrath of the male nurse reader. It would be impossibly clumsy if the nurse was continually referred to as 'he or she', so I have bowed to the numerical superiority of the female nurse and represented the nurse throughout the text in the feminine gender.

I have always thoroughly enjoyed my contact with the nursing profession and have learned a great deal from nurses' sharp-witted comments based on sound practical experience with people. I can only hope that the nurses who give this book their time and concentration will find in it some reward for their efforts.

In my writing of this book I am deeply indebted to many people. I would like to acknowledge the help given to me by my colleagues, Dr Freeman and Sister Rae, Tutor at Glasgow Royal Mental Hospital, whose comments have been of great value. I also owe a great deal to Miss Lamb whose encouragement and advice has improved the original manuscript beyond measure. In writing this material I have also come to recognize the extent to which my fundamental views have been influenced by Mr J. C. Raven, under whom I originally trained at the Crichton Royal, Dumfries. My thanks are also due to Miss M. McDonald and Mrs M. Strachan, who assisted in the typing, and Miss E. McGill, who has had much of the laborious work of checking and proof reading. In the cause of domestic peace, I would also like to acknowledge the help of my wife, who provided the grammatical accuracy.

Finally, I would like to acknowledge the inestimable assistance given to me by all nurses with whom I have had contact. In a sense this book is written by them as much as myself.

Glasgow,
1959

A. McGhie

Contents

Part One
The Development of Personality

This first section of the book will be devoted to the examination of personality development. We will discuss development in four separate chapters pertaining to the developmental stages of childhood, adolescence, adulthood, and old age. Our discussion in this section of the book will be more detailed and exhaustive than any later sections. There are two main reasons for placing so much emphasis on this part of our subject. There is first the practical reason which arises from the importance placed on personality development in the psychology course now offered to candidates for the General Nursing Council Examination. As the main aim of teaching psychology to nurses is to widen their understanding of human behaviour, it is also most important that the nurse has as full a conception as possible of the normal course of human development. The reader may find herself a little put off by a few of the psychological terms which face her, particularly at the beginning of this section. It will be found, however, that these terms are later described in more detail and illustrated by examples which, it is hoped, will make them more readily understood.

1. Childhood

The First Months

It has often been said, usually by rather bewildered fathers, that the child has no personality until around the second year of life and that one infant is very much the same as another. This view reflects the fact that the infant has not yet fully developed the distinctive ways of adjusting himself to his environment (the personality traits) which will later allow us to respond to him as a unique individual. Most mothers would, however, hotly deny such an assertion and point out that, from the first week of life, they have no difficulty in noticing aspects of behaviour which distinguish their infant from all other babies.

What is the actual inner world of the young infant? What, if anything, does he experience, and how much importance has this experience in shaping the infant's later life?

From a physiological viewpoint the infant's most striking characteristic is the lack of integration in its behaviour. The brain and nervous system are not yet fully developed and the sense organs are unco-ordinated and responsive to only intense stimuli. Surrounded by a mass of meaningless stimuli which are transmitted through the senses, the infant's world must indeed approach the 'booming, buzzing confusion' to which the psychologist, William James, likened it. It is only gradually, through frequent experience and repetition, that the infant learns to distinguish specific objects from the mass of stimuli surrounding it and to attach specific meanings to these objects. Thus such stimuli as the breast or feeding bottle, the sound of mother's voice, and parts of the infant's own body, become separated from the rest of the environment and come to have a meaning of their own. However, the most important object which the infant is gradually learning to distinguish from the outside world is its own self.

Adualism

One of the foremost names in the subject of infantile development is that of Jean Piaget (1928, 1932, 1951), and it was he who introduced the term 'adualism' to describe the basic factor which sets apart the stage of infancy from all other developmental stages. As adults we have no difficulty in making a clear-cut distinction between our thoughts, images, feelings—all that is internal and part of the self—and objects and events in the outside world. We are so accustomed to this state of mind where internal mentality and external reality are clearly distinguished that it is difficult for us to visualize any other form of existence. Yet the infant in the stage of 'adualism' has not yet attained this capacity. At this level there is no differentiation between the self and the outside world, no self-awareness, no consciousness of external objects. During infancy the child must learn to differentiate objects from its total background of experience and its first task is to form an idea of the self as an object distinct from other objects. This the infant does gradually through repeated experience. Anyone who has closely observed infants during the first six months of life will have seen how the infant ceaselessly explores its own body, gradually learning its own 'body boundaries.' In a similar process of trial and error the infant slowly learns the limits of its own 'mental boundaries' and begins to assert its own individuality in its relations with the objects which surround it.

The Infant's Relations with Others

The first year of life has provided a fertile field for psychological theories concerning the influence on the child of the behaviour of the adults around it. Many such theories have postulated that the infant is capable of complex thinking and is acutely sensitive to the effect of the relationships it forms with objects in its environment, particularly the mother. The work of Piaget and other investigators of infantile perceptual development tends to contradict these assumptions. In the initial state of adualism the infant is incapable of perceiving separate objects in its environment. It has been demonstrated that, even at a later stage when the infant is able to distinguish and recognize objects, the objects are not perceived as having a permanent existence. By permanence of the object we refer to the fact that we ordinarily perceive an object as having an independent existence even when it can no longer be perceived. To the young infant, however, the object only exists while it is actually present. If the object is taken away and re-presented later it will be recognized by the infant, but all experimental evidence suggests that, during the period in which the object is absent, the infant retains no memory image of the object. It is not until somewhere around the fifth to tenth month that the infant perceives the object as having a permanent and independent existence and it follows that, before this developmental stage is reached, the infant cannot form any permanent relationship with outside objects. The practical value of such a discovery is evident when we consider the mother or any other adult as the object in question for we must conclude that the child is incapable of forming any permanent relationship with the mother during the first six months of life. Certainly the infant may appear to disagree with our conclusion by its lusty and continual crying in mother's absence. There is, of course, no doubt that the infant becomes accustomed to the mother's personal ways of nursing and may be sensitive to any changes or irregularities in its general care and handling. It is, however, a far cry from recognizing the establishment of a physiological rhythm of this nature to speaking of the infant's emotional relationship with the mother. The common hospital practice of separating the infant from the mother immediately after birth apart from brief feeding periods has been frowned upon by many psychologists on the grounds that such separation interrupts the child's emotional attachment to the mother and thus predisposes the infant to acute anxiety. One could argue that such separation might have adverse effects on the mother who is denied the opportunity to accustom herself to handling the child but it would seem unlikely that the early separation has any effect on the newborn infant who probably is content to leave the anxiety to the psychologist. This is not to underestimate the importance of 'mothering' on the infant's development, for there seems little doubt that the infant's primitive nervous system does require such tactile stimulation and movement for its development. The criticism here is directed more towards the tendency to evolve a variety of authoritatively sounding theories regarding the early mother-child relationship which are in total contradiction to what little we do know of this early stage of life.

A good example of information derived by psychologists in recent studies of the infant's relations with others is given in Schaffer's (1961) study of 'attachment' behaviour at different stages in infancy. His work suggests that there are three separate phases in the development of the infant's attachment to other people. In the first stage, which occurs during the first three months of life, the infant's main need appears to be for a variety of sensory stimulation from its environment.

One of the pre-requisites of normal development during the first few months of life would appear to be that the infant is stimulated through its sense organs by a certain level of sensory stimuli. Thus it receives tactile stimuli through being handled by others and through its own movements. From its environment the infant also receives the constant stream of auditory and visual sensations which again appear to play a necessary part in developing his primitive nervous system. The important point of this first and early stage of *sensory stimulation* is that during this time the infant seeks stimulation in the form of any type of environmental change, rather than specifically social stimulation. Thus the young child of up to 3 months may cry if left alone in his pram, but be quite content when any sort of stimulation is introduced. Many mothers have indeed found the usefulness of such objects as vacuum cleaner, radio, or even television in satisfying the restless young infant. Between the third and seventh months of of life, a new phase in the development of social behaviour is reached which Schaffer describes as the phase of *indiscriminate social* attachment. During this period the normal infant shows a need to be stimulated by people, but his need is not discriminative in that it does not appear to be attached to any particular person. Thus, during this phase the child's crying may cease when he is approached by anybody, whether they be familiar to him or complete strangers. The 5-month-old infant left in his pram, for example, may cry when his mother leaves him to go into a shop, but he is likely to quieten down when any passer-by approaches and takes up his attention. This behaviour is in marked distinction to the later *discriminative social* stage of development which Schaffer has found does not occur until around the seventh month of life. The infant at this stage, if left alone in his pram, may not cease crying until the reappearance of his mother or some other familiar figure. Schaffer has also shown that usually, within a month after this stage has been reached, the child indicates clearly his ability to discriminate between people, by showing his first fear reaction to strangers. If we then accept that the infant's need for stimulation follows the three stages outlined by Schaffer, we can see that up to the age of 3 months the infant will respond favourably to any type of environmental stimulation, social or otherwise. From 3 to 7 months he will show a need for social stimulation, but this will be indiscriminate in the sense that he will respond equally well to any person. It is only after the age of 7 months that the child first begins to show a need for constant stimulation by one or a few selected people in his environment. Even after this stage, infants appear to vary a great deal in their need for physical contact involved in mothering. Some infants appear to crave a great deal of hugging, cuddling, kissing, and other such tactile stimulation, while others react more negatively to such stimulation. These latter infants may respond more favourably to what one might call 'non-contact' stimulation such as the sound of the mother's voice. Schaffer has suggested that mothers also show great individual differences in their need for physical contact with their infant and he suggests that the initial phase of mothering involves a great deal of mutual adaptation between mother and child. It may well be that some forms of disturbance shown by infants are due to a relationship involving opposites. One might visualize, for example, a mother who has a strong need for physical contact with her infant becoming distressed by an infant who shows a negative reaction to such stimulation. Other infants in turn who indicate a strong need for physical contact may become disturbed if the mother is herself unable or unwilling to supply this form of stimulation. The effect of a mother's behaviour upon the infant's development during the first year of life is a vast and interesting area which has remained almost completely neglected until recent years. Careful studies of the mother-child relationship in infancy, as carried out by Schaffer and others, tell a great deal about the many complex factors operating in early life, and also shed a little light on some of the disturbances which may occur in infancy as a reaction to hospitalization.

The subject of infant feeding has long provided a breeding ground for psychological theories which are so often unfortunately accepted as facts. In studying the infant's reactions to feeding we must preserve the same note of caution to prevent ourselves reading a meaning and significance into the infant's behaviour which is beyond his very limited repertoire during the first six months of life. Many words in the literature on child development have been devoted to the beneficial effects of breat-feeding as compared with bottle-feeding of the young infant. There is little doubt that natural breast-feeding may promote both physiological and psychological changes in the mother which are beneficial and that in this way the breast-feeding mother may gain relative to the bottle-feeding mother. However, many of the writers on this subject have postulated that breast-feeding is essential to the psychological development of the infant and that the bottle-fed baby is denied an important element in normal development. At various times it has been suggested that there is a connection between lack of breast-feeding and later personality developments such as delinquency and other disturbances of behaviour. The acceptance of the psychological importance to the infant of breat-feeding has led many hospitals to adopt an authoritarian and rigid approach to the nursing mother with resultant anxiety and guilt on the part of the mother who finds herself unable to cope with the role. It seems unlikely that the infant during the first six months of life experiences any differentiation between the breast and the bottle. From watching a hungry baby feeding one might conclude that the child's concern is with the contents rather than the container.

We have argued here than an active two-way relationship between mother and infant is, strictly speaking, impossible until the child has reached the stage of development where it becomes capable of relating itself to another person. At the same time we must not under-estimate the importance of the normal mother's way of reacting to her child as a complete 'person' from the beginning of its existence. The many normal aspects of mothering during these first months of the baby's life undoubtedly play an essential part not only in aiding the mother in adapting herself to the child but also in assisting the infant's gradual emergence of its own personality. It would surely be a mistake to endeavour, on the grounds of scientific accuracy, to explain to the new mother that her baby could not fully respond to her during its first six months. Fortunately, however, such explanation, even if it were given, would undoubtedly be scornfully rejected by most mothers.

Development of Thinking in Early Childhood

We have already discussed the young infant's emergence from the original state of adualism in which there is an absence of self-awareness. The development of self-awareness is a gradual process and it is not until the third or fourth year of life that it is completely achieved. This delay in development is probably due to a variety of factors. Although the young infant demonstrates some degree of memory in the first year of life observation shows that the memory process at first extends only to recognition and that recollection is not possible until the end of the first year. The infant may respond with joy to the reappearance of a favourite toy which he recognizes, but he cannot recall the toy in its absence. We have already seen that there are no permanent objects in the mind of the young infant. Later, during the second year of life when recollection becomes possible, it still covers only very short periods of time and remains very unstable until the third year. The young child, in fact, lives very much in the present, having little concern for the past and little awareness of the future. Since the idea of oneself and one's identity is, in a sense, an abstraction or a common factor of all one's personal memories it must obviously be retarded by the incomplete development of the memory processes. Another factor delaying the development of self-awareness is seen in the young child's lack of the necessary background of experience. It is only through repeated experiences involving such events as separation that the child can be allowed to build up a differential idea of himself as distinct from others.

Other psychological studies serve to remind us that the picture of the outside world which is transmitted through the senses of a young child may differ greatly from that gained by the older child and adult. For example, adequate perception of our environment is dependent, not only upon the functioning of the various senses but also upon our capacity to integrate this information into a meaningful pattern. If we go lower down the evolutionary scale it is evident that in many animals such integration is undeveloped. A frog will continue to respond to the visual stimulus of a fly by striking with its tongue even though each stroke results in the tongue being torn on sharp objects surrounding the fly. The information received from the tactile-pain sense is not integrated with the information received visually and behaviour remains unmodified and inefficient. A number of careful studies of younger children (e.g. Birch and Lefford, 1963) suggest a similar lack of integration of information received through different sensory modalities so that the child's perception of the inner world is more fragmentary. Such studies clearly illustrate how this kind of intersensory liaison gradually increases with age, greatly improving the child's perceptual development. The development of intersensory functioning is probably dependent upon both adequate maturation of the cerebral structures responsible for unifying different informational channels and repeated experience and practice with objects in the environment. Although a great deal of further research is required to define more clearly the effect of delayed intersensory organization upon the child's behaviour it is already evident from current studies that the acquisition of some skills, such as reading ability, are dependent upon adequate auditory-visual integration (Birch and Lefford, 1967).

A final drawback is the child's deficiency in language. His ideas expressing the relationship between himself and his environment are only dimly formed and can only become fully established with the further development of speech. A critical stage in the development of self-awareness appears to be reached around the age of 2 years and is marked by the period of *negativism* which most adults who have dealt with 2-year-old children will have no difficulty in recognizing. During this period the once relatively placid child becomes a rebellious and obstinate little tyrant whose one pleasure seems to be in doing exactly the opposite of what he is told and resisting all attempts to make him conform. It is as if the child, beginning to appreciate his own individuality, preserves and augments it by this demonstration of his own initiative and self-determination. In this way the negativistic period, although trying to adults around it, is probably essential to the child's normal mental development. A too severe restriction of the child's first bid for liberty at this time probably exerts a detrimental effect on the child's attainment of mental maturity.

Unlike rational adult thinking which is basically dependent upon a clear-cut distinction between the self and external reality, the child's thinking does not at first follow a set of logical rules which we assume to govern normal adult thinking. (As we shall see later, when we come to discuss adult thinking, this assumption is perhaps not quite as justified as we like to suppose.) The child's thinking, after it emerges from the primitive infantile state of adualism, has been termed 'egocentric' in so far as every experience, whether bodily or environmental, is viewed in terms of the self. Psychologists such as Piaget and Werner have attempted to illustrate the rules which govern egocentric thinking and which mark off this type of thinking from rational adult thinking which does not emerge until around the age of 8 years. A consideration of some of the main features of egocentric thought gives us a fuller insight into the mental life of the young child and perhaps a fuller understanding of the gulf which separates it from the adult view of the world.

Characteristics of Egocentric Thinking

In his thinking the young child is very much a confirmed egotist. His world is a limited one and he sees himself as the centre of it. Whereas in adult thinking we constantly alter our ideas to conform to reality the child rather distorts reality, moulding it to fit in with his own personal and subjective viewpoint. Let us now consider a few of the consequences of the child's prelogical egocentric type of thinking.

An analysis of children's speech during the egocentric phase reveals that for some time the young child feels no need to use his speech as a method of communication with others. The child's speech is often, in fact, a form of verbal thinking, and it is not until some time later that the child learns to think inwardly and silently. Although young children may appear to exchange information through speech, this rarely involves any modification of opinion. Indeed, the young child shows an almost complete disregard of the point of view of others, clinging with impressive tenacity to his own opinions. Perhaps most of us never completely outgrow this tendency. Exchange of information between children occurs later but still for some time such exchange involves no modification of opinion and the child still shows an inability to consider the viewpoint of others and to modify his own opinions accordingly.

Another demonstration of the egocentric nature of the child's thinking is seen in his difficulty in dealing with *conceptual* relations. The child may, for example, appear to understand the relationship between 'up' and 'down' and, in fact, use these terms correctly in his speech. However, the same child may become thoroughly confused when asked to accept that the stairs run 'up' when he is going upstairs to bed and run 'down' when he comes downstairs in the morning. The same difficulty arises with such relations as 'right' and 'left.' Before the age of 6 years the child displays a

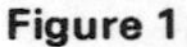

Figure 1

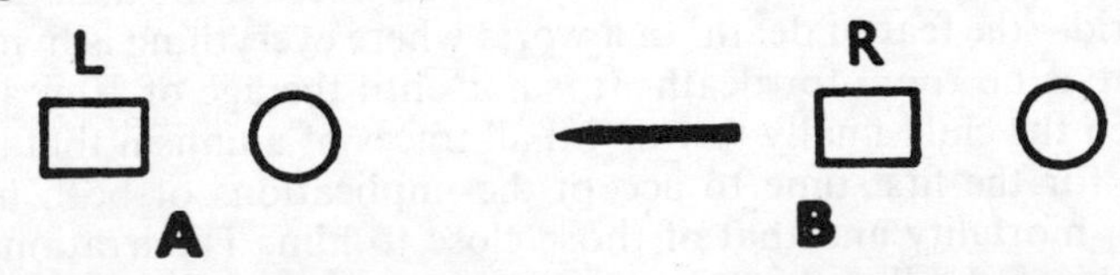

This little experiment demonstrates simply the young child's difficulty in dealing with spatial relations. In situation A he is presented with a ball and a building block and has little difficulty in seeing that the block is to the left of the ball. In situation B a pencil has now been placed at the other side of the block from the ball. The child cannot deduce that the block is now to the right of the pencil.

marked inability to appreciate the relations of 'right' and 'left' on his own body. From his egocentric viewpoint he cannot see why the positions should remain constant when he moves his body and will frequently be confused between his right and left hand. Somewhere around 6 years the child learns to differentiate correctly between right and left on his own body but still cannot correctly define these relations when applied to external objects or persons. His spatial relations are still subjectively centred around himself and it is not until nearer the 8th year that they become objective and the child perceives the relations objectively as independent of his own orientation.

A further consequence of the egocentric phase of development is that the child's world is essentially *animistic* or alive. To him there is no such thing as an inanimate object. He is living, therefore all other objects must also be alive. It is of interest to note that we as adults often encourage the child in his animistic viewpoint, finding it somehow attractive. Thus when the child falls and bangs his leg on a chair, mother is apt to say something like 'Bad chair to hit my little boy's leg.' Probably there are still traces of animism in our adult thinking as evidenced by such phrases as 'a threatening sky,' 'a cheerful looking fire,' and so on. Later the child learns that all objects in the world are not alive but still believes that all moving things are alive. Walking along a road one day in autumn with my own son, at that time aged 3½, a passing bus caused the leaves aligning the gutter to blow across in front of our path. My son, noting this event asked, 'Why do the leaves run away; are they frightened of the bus?' An appreciation of the animistic nature of the child's world aids one in understanding many childhood fears which seem quite resistant to the rational explanations offered to the child by adults. A world where every object is imbued with life must indeed at times be a rather fearful one. Animism does, however, hide from the child one source of fear which does haunt the adult world—the fear of death. In a world where everything is living there is no room for death. It is not until the age of 10 years when the child finally throws off all traces of animism that he has for the first time to accept the implications of both his own mortality and that of those close to him. The irrational world of childhood is given up only at some cost.

All investigations of children's thinking indicate that it is not until the age of approximately 8 years that the child is capable of the logical conceptual thinking associated with adult thought processes. It would be wrong, however, to assume that the young child is wholly incapable of any form of concept formation. Early in his development, in fact, we can observe the formation of *primitive concepts* which are based on a logic different from that used in adult conceptual thinking. Let us take a few illustrative examples. The objects which constitute the world of the child are essentially fused with the child's actions, their meaning and significance being in terms of the extent to which the child can use them in action. The child's primitive concept of 'a door' may include not only doors but boxes, drawers, and, in fact, any object which may be opened. His concept of 'a car' may extend to any object which can be pushed along the ground. Thus the child forms concepts but they often bear little relationship to the more objective concepts characteristic of adult thinking. The child's attempts to form his primitive concepts often provide amusing results. Some time ago my own child was introduced to the 'potty' in a half-hearted attempt to encourage him in toilet-training. It was one of the modern type shaped like a duck complete with duck's head. Within a few days my son had formed a primitive concept of this new object 'a potty' and could be found performing his functions on or in all his toys which resembled ducks. Being a psychologist I solved the problem with great subtlety by knocking the duck's head off the receptacle. However, my son was not to be deterred so easily and his next primitive concept had more tragic repercussions. One would assume that he now formed a concept of 'a potty' around any hollowed-out object of a roughly spherical shape for, a week later, he extended my limits of parental patience by eliminating the contents of his bladder in my best hat.

A final characteristic of egocentric thinking is demonstrated in the child's confusion between internal images and symbols on the one hand and external events and objects on the other. Although no longer bound by the phase of adualism which dominates the major part of the first year of development, the child still has a very tenuous hold on the difference between internal mental processes and external events. Thus a child finds it difficult to understand why others cannot see his dreams if they are in the room with him while he sleeps. The child considers the dream, an internal image, as being an externally located event observable by others. But this confusion is not confined to the dream state. In waking life the child frequently fails to differentiate clearly between his own inner images and thoughts and 'real' events in the outside world. In everyday life we refer to the child's 'vivid imagination' to describe his tendency to confuse reality with phantasy. However, the child's 'imaginings' are of a different order from the day-dreaming of the adult for the child is often genuinely unable to differentiate between the two. The little boy who breaks one of his mother's dishes only to protest with wide-eyed innocence that 'It was a little man who came in the window and did it' may be punished for telling a lie. In actual fact, the child may himself believe his tale and regard the subsequent punishment as a severe injustice. The confusion between thought and reality may result in the child often only having to think something to be convinced of its external reality. We refer to the *omnipotence of thought* to describe the all-powerful, almost magical nature of thinking at this stage of development. Thoughts and the words which express them have to the child an independent and objective existence. I remember a father telling me how his young daughter was terrified of his tape recorder which she feared would 'take away my words and keep them shut up in that box.'

We might conclude from this consideration of egocentric thinking that the 'laws' which govern it are in many ways quite different from the logical rules of later adult thinking. Obviously the development of adult thinking is dependent upon the presence and gradual integration of organic cerebral structures. At the same time the observations of students of child development have indicated that 'logical thinking is necessarily social.' It is only in his constant interactions with others that the child becomes more free of the original egocentrism and thus able to establish mature socialized reciprocal relations between himself and others.

Egocentric Thinking and Adult Mental Disorders

In the face of severe stress adults may often show childlike reactions (see discussion on 'Regression', Chapter 6). When the adult suffers from an actual mental disorder this resemblance between adult and childhood behaviour is often very striking and knowledge of the egocentric thinking of the child may help us in understanding the behaviour of the sick adult. Adult patients with a neurotic disorder often display childlike qualities, particularly in the emotionally uncontrolled nature of their behaviour. It is, however, in the behaviour of the more seriously disordered psychotic patient that we find the closest correspondence with the egocentric child. A progressive loss of distinction between fantasy and reality is one of the most characteristic features of schizophrenia (to be considered in more detail in the next chapter). The adult schizophrenic constantly projects on to external reality his own inner wishes, fears and thoughts, resulting in the same type of reality distortion seen in early childhood. The omnipotence of thoughts already described may be found in the adult patient who feels others can see the thoughts in his head or that people are taking his words away from him while he speaks. Traces of animistic thinking, dormant since early childhood, may again appear so that a patient imbues life and direction to inanimate objects and non-human creatures. Like the young child he may perceive and interpret events around him solely from his own perspective. In the more extreme and advanced stages of an illness the patient may show the same inability to differentiate between the self and the remainder of the environment as found in the adualistic phase of early infancy. In his condition, he may show frequent confusions of identity, when his personality appears to merge with that of others around him. Some psychoanalysts think that the adult patient regresses to a more primitive level of mental functioning because of his inability to adjust to the demands of adult life. Implicit in this point of view is the idea that patients who later develop such an illness had a particularly traumatic early childhood which renders later mature adjustment impossible. Regression in this sense means that the adult patient is pulled back to a more primitive mode of adjustment by the unresolved conflicts of childhood. However, the correspondence between childhood and adult mental illness may be interpreted in a rather different manner. An adult patient with a severe brain injury may show many regressive components in his behaviour in so far as he behaves in a childlike way. The main reason for such regression is that the injury has impaired his adult higher mental functions and caused him to function at a lower level. Many psychiatrists who regard severe mental disorders such as schizophrenia as being organic in origin, argue that the patient regresses in his behaviour not because of early unresolved infantile conflicts but because the illness causes damage to the brain and nervous system. In this view the regressed patient is not so much pulled back to an earlier more primitive level of adjustment but is rather pushed back by his current condition.

Although the similarities between psychotic adult behaviour and normal childhood behaviour have been emphasized there are numerous differences. While the resemblances are useful in helping to understand the behaviour of the psychotic patient this should not lead us to treat a patient as a child. No matter how severe the illness or how destructive it is to the adult personality, the patient still retains some residue of adult functioning.

The Emotional Life of the Child

Thus far we have been primarily concerned with the child's mental development and we have rather neglected the emotional side of childhood development. Any distinction between these two aspects of the child's personality is obviously artificial as they are interdependent, but for explanatory purposes it is useful to consider emotional development in a separate section.

Psycho-analytic theory regards the emotional reactions formed in childhood as all-important in so far as they form the basis of the adult personality and it is to psycho-analytic investigations that we owe a great deal of our conceptions of early emotional development. Freud (1923) referred to the child's life being directed by the *pleasure principle* in that it is dominated by powerful emotional drives. These drives are characterized by their lack of control and their need to obtain immediate satisfaction. Gradually, through contact and repeated experience with the outside world, the child learns to conform to social demands and to control and, if necessary, delay the satisfaction of his primitive emotional drives. The child now ceases to live entirely for the moment and learns to appreciate the future consequences of his actions and to adapt himself to the external world. In psychoanalytic terminology the child now adapts to the *reality principle*. The source of the original strong and primitive drives is termed the *Id* (Unconscious) whereas the subsequent emergence of a more socialized self is termed the *Ego* (Conscious). The gradual emotional development in childhood, then, consists of the processes of the ego gradually gaining ascendance over the forces of the id. Emotional maturity is, then, attained when the child learns to reject the pleasure principle and to adopt the reality principle in his dealings with his environment. For some time, however, the child's life is still dominated by the primitive drives behind the reality principle. There is an obvious similarity between this psycho-analytic concept of early development and the sequence, already outlined, of adualism emerging into egocentric thought and finally, under environmental pressures, being resolved into mature rational thinking. The main difference in the two approaches, apart from the terminology, is that the psycho-analytic system stresses the emotional side of development while the genetic approach is more concerned with intellectual development.

One of the first emotional crises which the child faces is the resolution of the *Oedipus Complex*. This much maligned psychoanalytic term merely seeks to denote the stage of childhood development (occurring about the age of 4) at which the child forms an increasingly possessive and demanding emotional bond with the parent of the opposite sex with corresponding feelings of jealousy and aggression towards the parent of the same sex and, in fact, towards any other individuals who come between the child and the parent. In the normal child evidence of this attitude disappears by about the fifth year, by which time the child has begun to *identify* itself with the parent of the same sex. Such identification may be seen as the child's first stage in the process of development towards his expected social role.

The relatively uncontrolled nature of the child's emotional reactions means that feelings at this phase of development are uninhibited. Anyone who has witnessed the reaction of a child to a situation which refuses gratification of his wants will readily agree to the intensity of the emotions. We need, in fact, look no farther than the 3-year-old or 4-year-old child for an illustration of the full force and depth of our emotions. The child's feelings, which are unaffected by considerations of reason or consequence, govern his actions. Some time ago I attended a meeting of a children's 'court of law,' formed in a child guidance clinic to encourage self-responsibility and self-government in the group of children. The 'accused' in this case was a boy who had been caught stealing from his fellows. In my innocence I wondered why the adults in charge did not leave the whole procedure entirely in the hands of the children. Subsequent events soon made the reason for adult control apparent. The boy was found guilty by the 'jury' of children who, when asked to decide on appropriate punishment, responded with the cry of 'Let's hang him!'

The child lives in a simple black and white world, uncluttered by intermediate shades of grey. He hates and loves with a passionate fervour although his passion may change from one moment to the next. Often his feelings are *ambivalent* in that he feels the opposite emotions of love and hate at the same time towards the same object. He loves his parents, upon whom he is wholly dependent, but at times they frustrate him in his desires, and he responds with feelings of hate and aggression. The primitive and spontaneous nature of the young child's emotional reactions led a psychological colleague specializing in work with children to remark, half seriously, 'Perhaps child psychology should really be a branch of zoology.' The development and subsequent control of the emotions in childhood, like all other aspects of development, does not exist in a vacuum but within the framework of the child's relationship with others. The most important relationships the child makes are, of course, with its parents and so we obtain a greater understanding of emotional development by observing the child in the family situation.

The Child and the Family

One of the many factors which separate man from all other animals is the long period of development which occurs before complete maturity and self-dependence can be reached. The child's greatest need during its development is for a feeling of security which stems from an awareness of being wanted and loved by the adults upon whom he depends. The idea we form of ourself and our self-esteem depends in great measure upon the picture of ourself which we see reflected in the eyes of those around us. A child who is continually derided by his parents as being stupid and clumsy may well grow up with this image of himself indelibly printed in his mind. The child's early environment is a limited one and his view of the world and his own place in it will be shaped mainly by his relationship with his family. During infancy and early childhood the most important figure is obviously the mother who is constantly with the child catering to his many needs. Because of this, most studies of the young child in the family have concentrated on the mother-child relationship. As usual we appear to know more of what constitutes an unsatisfactory mother-child relationship than we do of the factors involved in an ideal relationship. Let us here consider three types of mother-child relationship which, each in their own way, can be seen as detrimental to the child's stable development.

The child may be *rejected* by the mother. Here we do not refer to the actual physical rejection of an unwanted baby but to an emotional rejection. In this relationship the child's basic needs may be catered for but in a mechanical affectionless manner, the mother responding to the child as an object rather than a living being. The picture of a mother who is unable to accept and love her child is a familiar one to those engaged in the treatment of childhood maladjustment. We might expect such a child to grow up to be emotionally blunted in his capacity to respond to or accept affection from others. The opposite, but equally harmful, type of relationship is seen in the case of the child who is *over-protected* by the mother. Although the child must be protected to some extent from dangers in the environment, we have already seen that normal development demands that the child enjoy sufficient freedom to develop his own individuality. The over-protected child is denied this right to assert his own initiative and develops not as a separate person, but almost as an extension of the over-protecting mother. Although over-protection may apparently stem from excessive love on the part of the mother its true source invariably lies in the mother's inability to accept and love her child while respecting his right to grow up as an independent being. Such children tend to develop as emotionally immature, shy, and withdrawn adults who retain throughout life their need for dependency. One such adult described the source of her difficulties to the author with the apt comment: 'I wasn't mothered, I was smothered!' A third type of harmful relationship is when the mother's attitude towards her child is neither one of rejection nor over-protection but is predominantly *erratic*. In this setting the child is alternately loved or rejected according to the mother's prevailing mood. At one time his actions will be tolerated or even encouraged by mother while, at another time, the same behaviour will result in disapproval and punishment. The child subjected to the insecurity of this relationship will be equally hampered in his development and may, in later life, show a corresponding lack of self-confidence and mistrust of others. There is little doubt that each of the three relationships we have described is detrimental to healthy and stable development. However, we cannot afford to be too emphatic regarding their specific effects on later personality. It is only too easy to theorize regarding the probable outcome of such situations but what work has been done on the actual follow-up of cases to check specific effects on later personality indicates that human nature is infinitely complex and that the predictive value of such knowledge is anything but clear. We will see this same problem repeated again and again in problems involving human development. The original source of personality traits seems only too obvious when we look back over an adult's life, listening particularly to his early experiences as a child. However, when we try to apply our information in predicting future outcome on the basis of our knowledge of psychological factors now in operation in the child, we are often chastened to find that the expected pattern does not develop. The forces influencing and shaping the individual personality are manifold and it is difficult and dangerous to isolate one small segment of human experience as alone deciding the final product.

This conclusion is equally applicable when we consider the effects on the child of actual *separation* from the mother. A great deal has been written on the effects of separation from the mother during the first five years of life. Various investigations on this subject have suggested that such separation is not only detrimental to the child at the time of the separation but that the child may suffer from long-term effects which leave a permanent mark on the personality and on the individual's mental health. Most of the evidence for this view was summarized in this country by Bowlby (1951) whose name has become closely linked with the study of maternal deprivation. Later Bowlby and his colleagues (1956) reported a carefully controlled and detailed study of the personality differences existing between children who had suffered prolonged maternal separation (due to a tubercular illness requiring sanatorium treatment) during the first five formative years of life and children who were not thus deprived. The most important aspects of Bowlby's findings are described in the following extract from his report:'. . . it is clear that some of the former group of workers, including the present senior author, in their desire to call attention to dangers which can often be avoided have on occasion overstated their case. In particular, statements implying that children who are brought up in institutions or who suffer other forms of serious privation and deprivation in early life commonly develop psychopathic or affectionless characters are seen to be mistaken. . . . Outcome is immensely varied, and of those who are damaged only a small minority develop those very serious disabilities of personality which first drew attention to the pathogenic nature of the experience' (Bowlby, 1956). Some differences between the two groups were observed but it is difficult to ascertain the extent to which they are related to maternal separation as opposed to the many other variables which divide the two groups. All that we may conclude is that, although separation in childhood is undesirable, its effects on later personality are difficult to assess and have possibly been exaggerated by many reports.

The Role of the Father

Thus far we have been stressing the child's relationship with his mother and it may be thought we have forgotten that the child has also a father. In infancy and early childhood the father is usually rather out of the picture. Perhaps one day someone will make a study of the rejected father rather than the rejected child. In later childhood, however, the father's role gains in importance as the child becomes less dependent on his mother. Particularly in the case of the male child the establishment of a satisfactory relationship with the father is imperative for normal development, for it is through his *identification* with his father and his desire to be like him that the little boy adopts the characteristics of the male role. One of the main patterns of behaviour which boys learn through identification with their father is in the handling of their own aggressive drives. One might expect, then, that in homes where the father is absent during the child's early development, the male child is likely to be delayed in the emergence of his aggressive behaviour. The effect of a father's absence on the development of male children has been investigated by a number of psychologists (*e.g.* Sears *et al.*, 1946) who have compared children from homes where the father is present throughout development with those whose father has been separated from the home by such factors as military service. These studies indicate that the father's absence has a considerable effect in hampering the boy's personality development, while this influence is not apparent in the case of girls. This is as one would expect since girls are expected to identify with their mother. There is also some evidence to suggest that if the male child is unable to identify with his father, there is a greater likelihood of the emergence of pathological and delinquent behaviour in later years. A father to a young boy represents his first authority figure and his later attitude to authority in general may, to a great extent, be based on the factors operating in this original relationship. As the child develops he normally assigns to his father the role of an all-knowing superman who represents the child's ideal. The father's reign of king of the universe is, however, relatively short-lived for, as we shall see later, in the adolescent period he is usually toppled from his throne in favour of new heroes. Later in life the normal individual learns to accept a more realistic estimation of his father which lies between the uncritical hero-worship of childhood and the rebellious rejection of adolescence. This sequence of events in the child's relationship with his father is well summarized in the following remark which was made by a friend's son to his mother: 'You know it's a funny thing! When I was ten I used to think that father knew everything. When I was fifteen I thought father knew nothing, and now when I am twenty I find myself thinking what a lot father has learned in the last five years.'

Sibling Rivalry

The child's horizon cannot forever be limited to his relations with his parents. He has to learn to adjust himself to others and in his play with other children he learns more of the 'give and take' of life. The play situation presents another socializing influence in so far as the child has to adapt himself to the demands and rules of conduct set by other children. However, most children are forced to adjust themselves to this situation at an earlier age, inside the family circle, by virtue of the presence of brothers and sisters who also make demands on the parents. It is in his interactions with his siblings that the child is often introduced to his first competitive situation. Not only charity, but democracy, begins at home! The child's reactions to his siblings will, of course, depend a great deal upon the way in which his parents handle the situation. At the same time, even the most thoughtful of parents cannot prevent some degree of rivalry arising among the children in the family. Some measure of competition and rivalry is indeed inherent in the situation and probably exerts a healthy influence on the child's development, preparing him for the knocks he will later have to take in the less sheltered world outside the home. In a healthy home the child will soon learn to adapt his demands and needs to those of his siblings and benefit from their companionship. Unfortunately, the attitude of the parents may interfere with this adjustment and exaggerate the rivalry in the situation. Children are individuals and as such display different characteristics which may make them less or more endearing to adults. This is particularly the case with children at different age levels. The cute youngster of 2 years may no longer appear so attractive at the ripe age of 8 years. All parents will agree that there should be no favourites in the family but it is harder to put this maxim into practice and children are only too sensitive to any indications of partiality on the part of the parents. Naturally, a new member of the family demands more of the mother's time and care and the child who has so far enjoyed a monopoly of affection must feel somewhat displaced. If the mother can encourage the child to 'help' her in looking after the new baby and the father aids by spending more time with the child, the sharp edge of rejection may be removed from the situation. Again, it is impossible to prevent the child feeling some aggression towards the new child and for some time such feelings can be clearly observed. A mother once related to me how one morning she had run out of firewood and had asked her young 3-year-old son what they could use to light the fire. The reply was immediate and emphatic: 'Baby brother!'

In many cases the most traumatic feature to the child of the sibling situation is its manner of introduction. It is now more common for the mother during her pregnancy to prepare the child for the subsequent appearance of the new arrival but one still finds families where the whole situation is deliberately shrouded in mystery. An adult patient, who had been 8 years old when his sister was born, once told me: 'The one thing I remember about the birth of my sister was the whispering and secrecy. There was so much of it that I suspected something terribly evil and catastrophic must be about to happen.' Even the well-prepared child often has to suffer the double discomfort and shock of separation from the mother when she enters hospital and her return with the new member of the family.

In spite of the complications we have discussed the fact remains that most children learn to adapt themselves to the changed situation and later benefit from the companionship of their siblings. A great deal has been written regarding the more harmful effects on the child of having no siblings and we tend to have a stereotyped picture of the only child, spoiled, selfish, and lonely. This need not necessarily be true but obviously the only child is denied not only the companionship of siblings but the very useful corrective training which their presence brings. Perhaps once again, however, it is the parents who suffer more than the child for they may tend to become over-attached and over-dependent on their one child who, in the natural course of development, must some day break the bond to lead his own life independent of his parents.

Child Training

In modern times the psychologist and child psychiatrist have tended to become the high priests of child-rearing, their views often being adopted by doctors, nurses, welfare workers, and others who act in an advisory capacity to parents. This development is perhaps more obvious in the United States where the population appears to be more psychologically minded. In recent years in our own country there has been a growing tendency for parents to bring their children up 'by the book,' the 'book' being usually based upon psychological principles. As parents have grown more conscious of this form of guidance the books on this subject have vastly increased. Many a bewildered mother, faced with an embarrassing fund of contradictory information and advice, has returned to the adage that 'It's all a matter of common sense, anyway.' The systematic study of child development with its attempt to understand the mental processes of the child has been most productive and has vastly expanded our knowledge of a hitherto little known field and it would indeed be tragic if the fruits of such study were not incorporated into the actual practice of child-rearing. Unfortunately, however, many of the theories which have been put forward as fact have not been based on systematic study and, as a result, there has been a great deal of nonsense written on this subject which does psychology as a whole a great discredit and often causes concern and confusion in the minds of parents and others working with children. In the United States of America, for example, great stress has been placed on the correct timing of weaning and the dangerous effects of early or late weaning on later personality development although we really know very little regarding the long-term effects of weaning. Research studies as have been made have produced conflicting results. In the investigation carried out by Rogerson (1939), children who had been bottle-fed in infancy were found to be more neurotic in later life and to have a poorer school record. In contrast to this finding, several investigators (Peterson and Spano, 1941; Sewell and Mussen, 1952) failed to find any relationship between type of feeding and later personality development. Investigators have also suggested that the physical advantages of breast-feeding to the nursing mother and baby have been over-emphasized. A carefully conducted study of 106 nursing mothers in the Aberdeen area (Hytten *et al.*, 1958) recently indicated that 'It is quite clear that both mothers and babies did better with bottle-feeding. The bábies cried less, put on more weight, and were at least as healthy; and the mothers, apart from escaping trouble with breasts and nipples, were less tired.' The main difficulty, in the investigators' opinion, is that breast-feeding may tend to put excessive demands on a mother who, in our modern society, already has to cope with a great deal of strain. Their final conclusion is that 'We should help in every way possible the woman who wishes to breast-feed, but we are not justified in putting pressure on those who are unwilling or who appear to be unable to breast-feed efficiently' (Hytten *et al.*, 1958). Whatever the medical opinion of the relative merits or demerits of breast-feeding it is evident that the modern mother is moving away from natural feeding. It has been estimated that only one-third of mothers are now to be found breast-feeding after the third month.

One of the first traditional milestones in training with which the child has to cope is, of course, that of toilet training. Mothers are often advised by hospitals and clinics to commence toilet training almost immediately, while most of the accepted psychological books on child-rearing advise against this practice. In actual fact there is no possibility of the child achieving any form of voluntary control over his toilet functions during the first year of life as the necessary physiological apparatus is not yet established. By regular and repeated 'potting,' however, the mother may be able to establish a simple reflex response in which the stimulus of the pot automatically initiates the correct response. It would probably be more true to say that in most cases of early toilet training the child trains the mother rather than the reverse in so far as the mother learns to time her potting activity with the child's natural excretory rhythm. The chief dangers of early toilet training are twofold. A simple reflex response may be established during the first year which gives the appearance that the child has some degree of control over his functions. Somewhere around the age of 14 months, when the average child begins to attain a true voluntary control over his bladder and bowel functions, the whole process may well break down. Up to this point a simple habit has been established which, on the part of the child, is purely involuntary so that the child is quite likely to revolt against this habit-pattern once he has become aware of his ability to control his own functions. Although this breakdown in the established pattern of training may be only a temporary one the mother may become anxious and her attempts to discipline the child may well result in a more prolonged period of disturbance. The other, and perhaps more insidious, danger is that some mothers feel compelled to establish toilet training in the early months through an inherent disgust and abhorrence of the child's normal excretory functions. If this attitude on the part of the mother is exaggerated it may well have repercussions on later personality development, establishing in the child an unhealthy preoccupation with, and an aversion to, his normal bodily functions. The psycho-analysts believe that this type of traumatic toilet training may result in a later personality which is abnormally obsessional and over-concerned with such matters as cleanliness, general hygiene, and in establishing a sense of order. It is again probably dangerous to generalize in this way from one specific situation but, nevertheless, it is obviously undesirable that the child should grow up to regard his own normal bodily functions as repellent. Children learn most of their habits naturally and spontaneously through their identification with people around them, particularly their parents. In the normal course of development, then, the child somewhere during the course of his second year will indicate his readiness for toilet training in so far as he wishes to behave in the same way as his parents and siblings. Anthony (1957) has suggested that the optimum age for the beginning of toilet training is around 15 months for this is the age where the average child indicates his desire to literally 'follow in his father's footsteps.' At whatever the age training is begun the most important factor is the form which the training takes. Early training which is based on patience and tolerance on the part of the mother will obviously be a great deal less damaging than training which is not only early but severe and rigid.

It is by now a standard joke that the children of psychologists and other workers in this field are invariably undisciplined and insufferable little horrors. This conception is based on the stereotyped idea that psychologists advocate that the child be allowed to develop in complete freedom and that he be allowed to express himself without the restrictions of adult discipline. This, of course, is a complete misconception although the public cannot be held altogether responsible for its origin. It is certainly, as we have already argued, vitally important that the child be allowed to express his own personality and to attain a healthy and independent sense of his own initiative and self-determination. On the other hand, the child does look to the adults around him for guidance and for the establishment of a set of rules which will create some order in an otherwise chaotic world. Discipline in its correct sense should provide a necessary socializing force and prepare the child for his subsequent role as a member of human society. A complete lack of discipline is perhaps as harmful to the child as too much discipline. Sometimes the question of discipline hinges more specifically on the advisability or non-advisability of the application of physical punishment. There is little doubt that it would be ideal if all parents could provide an adequate training discipline for their children without recourse to spanking or any other form of physical chastisement. However, the ideal adult exists only as an abstraction and we must come down to earth when we are dealing with mere mortals such as ourselves. The author's experience of homes where any form of physical punishment was taboo is that the resultant tension and anxiety on the part of the parents can often have a more harmful effect on the child than a hand applied in the proper place at the proper time. However, as we have already seen, one's experience can be most misleading and once again it might be worth while for us to consider briefly some of the more objective studies that have been carried out on the effects of different types of parental discipline. Of the many studies that have been made in this field, that reported by Symonds (1939) is perhaps most representative in its findings. Symonds compared children from strict and authoritarian homes with children who were brought up in a more permissive atmosphere. He found that children reared by parents who were strict and rather restrictive in their attitude tended to be more obedient and courteous in their attitude to elders but at the same time were inclined to be very timid and socially withdrawn. The children of permissive parents tended on the other hand, to be less obedient, more aggressive, but at the same time were more secure, self-confident, and independent in their adjustment to life. Another interesting finding emerged from the research work of Shoben (1949) who compared a group of 'problem' children with a control group of 'non-problem' children. The former group were mainly delinquent or had been referred to Child Guidance Authorities for maladjusted behaviour. Shoben found that the parents of these problem children tended to adopt a strict disciplinary attitude and put a high premium on obedience in the home. In contrast to this, the children who displayed no deviant social behaviour tended to come from a home where parents were remarkedly less strict, more permissive, and more willing to tolerate their child developing independence in his behaviour. There are many other studies one could mention in this context but their findings point in general in the same direction. They suggest that strict training tends to be successful in producing a child who is obedient and who conforms readily to authority, but who is, however, at the same time less independent, more passive, and socially withdrawn. A more relaxed and permissive parental attitude tends, on the other hand, to produce a child who is somewhat more aggressive and less obedient but who gains by being more independent and better adjusted in his social life.

The Child's Moral Sense

As adults our conduct is still to some extent controlled by external authority. A stronger, and often more exacting, source of moral discipline is, however, represented by the internal 'voice of conscience.' Observation of child behaviour allows us some understanding of the mode of development of the child's moral sense which again appears as part of the whole socialization process rather than a naturally operating capacity. A 'conscience,' in the adult sense of an internal 'censor' guiding each individual's behaviour, does not appear to operate in the child until somewhere between the age of 5 and 7 years. Prior to this age the child is *amoral* in so far as he has no conception of an inherent right or wrong. He may well conform to a set of rules laid down by the disciplining adult but he does not accept these rules as comprising an inner code of conduct. To the young child at this stage wrong actions are simply these which are punished. By the age of 7 years the normal child incorporates within his own personality the restrictions of external authority thus marking the birth of the 'conscience,' an inner moral sense. 'Bad' behaviour is no longer that which carries a threat of punishment but also that which will result in the child 'feeling' bad. The child begins to appreciate that 'no man is an island' and that his actions affect others. He learns to do unto others as he would have done to himself and he becomes aware of shame and guilt as a consequence of ignoring his moral standards. It is perhaps interesting to note here that depressive illnesses, although much commoner than we might suppose in childhood, are not reported under the age of 7 years. One might also view the anti-social and delinquent older child as one who has not managed to negotiate this important step of internalizing a set of moral standards and who still associates a 'wrong' action merely with the possibility of external punishment.

Another source of stress to the young child may occur where the adults around him expect the child to appreciate the same moral principles as themselves. Children have great difficulty in understanding why their moralistic view of the world is so often at variance with that of their parents who condemn them for transgressing ethical boundaries which are beyond their comprehension. One of the best illustrations of the child's moralistic viewpoint is contained in the story of the Sunday School teacher who showed to her class of young children pictures illustrating scenes in ancient times when Christians were being thrown to the lions in view of their beliefs. The teacher was moved to find one of the little boys visibly distressed and near to tears, and hastened to reassure him. The little boy, however, burst into tears declaring earnestly—'But, teacher, that little lion there hasn't got a Christian.'

The fact that most children develop a moral sense by the age of 7 years does not, of course, mean that their moral standards will be necessarily similar. If these standards are founded originally as an incorporation of parental standards then of course individuals will vary in the content of their conscience. If the parents themselves are controlled by a rigid and harsh set of moral principles then the child may have his own personality permanently crippled by a conscience which is unnecessarily and unhealthily severe and over-demanding. A lack of moral values in the parents may also have a detrimental effect on the child in a different way although, in this situation, the child may still be able to learn his moral standards from the influence of others at a later age.

Another characteristic of moral behaviour is the capacity to deny the overt expression of certain impulses in behaviour. We can readily observe the young child's comparative inability to control his own responses. He acts on impulse, translating his feelings and desires into immediate action. One of the indications that the child is growing up and acting in a more controlled and adult manner is the emergence of the capacity to inhibit behavioural responses that have been up to now freely expressed. The developing child gradually learns to appreciate that his behaviour has an impact on others and that to find his place in the social group he has to constantly modify his behaviour to fit in with the rest of the group. The emergence of this type of more controlled and directed behaviour is gradual and its initiation and subsequent development varies greatly between different children. These individual differences naturally reflect differences in the general life situation of each individual child. There are some children however who appear to suffer from a developmental lag in this aspect of their behaviour, in that they remain impulsive, and apparently less able than others of their age to control their responses to the environment. Although developing normally in most other ways, such children remain unpredictable, antisocial, and explosive in their social behaviour. Such characteristics render them less well adapted to society and more likely to run into trouble with authority. We might expect children with such behavioural difficulties to be found with relatively high frequency in the populations of approved schools, borstals, and other corrective establishments. There is some experimental work which suggests that such failure to develop the capacity to inhibit response, which is a feature of normal social behaviour, may sometimes be a result of constitutional impairment resulting from minimal brain damage occurring at birth. The Russian psychologist Luria (1961) has developed experimental techniques for measuring the child's capacity to inhibit responses, and has used these to isolate groups of children who show an abnormal retardation in this aspect of their development. In this country, Tizard (1962) has applied similar techniques to groups of school children of different ages in order to trace changes in response inhibition with age. Tizard's work also suggests that children who do poorly on experimental tests of response inhibition tend to have more behavioural difficulties and to be generally more impulsive in their behaviour. This connection has been confirmed by the work of Lowe (1966) who, using similar techniques, has recently examined the relationship between response inhibition and socially deviant behaviour. One of the techniques here is to face the child with two types of simple stimuli (*e.g.* a bell and a buzzer). He is taught to respond to one of these stimuli by pressing a sensitized hand-trigger and to inhibit response to the alternative 'negative' stimulus. The two stimuli are then presented in a mixed series at different speeds of presentation, and the child's response examined. For most children beyond the age of 7, this is a relatively simple task which they carry out with very few errors. Some children, however, perform the task very badly, showing a repeated inability to inhibit their response to the negative stimulus. When descriptions and ratings of the child's social behaviour made by teachers are examined, it is found that the children who fail to respond adequately in such a test situation tend to be described as unusually impulsive, antisocial, and maladjusted in their behaviour. These children appear to have a genuine difficulty in controlling their own responses. It would be interesting to know what proportion of such children become deviant, delinquent or criminal in their adult behaviour.

The Child at School

Somewhere around the age of 5 years the child is called upon to adjust himself to a new situation—that of starting school. Once again we probably under-estimate the adaptability of the average child and the beginning of schooldays is often an event which is more traumatic to the mother than the child. Nevertheless, this does mark, for many children, the first real step completely outside the security and protection of the family and it must involve some measure of stress. In school the child must learn to be one of a group and to find his own role within that group. From my own schooldays I remember a boy who was ignored by the other children until he found that he could make others laugh at him playing the fool. He soon became the class clown and retained this role not only throughout his schooldays but into adult life. Others may find their place in the limelight by virtue of their physical prowess, their organizing ability, their appearance, or even by their nuisance value to the teacher. Our schools may not be 'blackboard jungles' but they are certainly often more elemental and primitive societies than the secure confines of the family circle.

The principal purpose of school is, however, not to give the child his first lesson in group psychology but merely to give him his first lesson. Here the child will have his first experience of formal learning and this experience may shape his whole future attitude to education. The true role of the primary school is then to provide an atmosphere which will be conducive to developing a healthy attitude to later learning. This view of early schooling is also supported by the fact that, at the age when he first starts school, the child's thinking and behaviour are still greatly under the control of the prelogical egocentric principles which we have already discussed. It is not until around the age of 7 or 8 years that children can be expected to begin to think in a logical manner and thus an appeal to rational learning at an earlier age is hardly likely to be successful. Many modern schools recognize the specialized function of the first years of schooling and, often under the fire of the fierce criticism of parents, aim simply at fostering a positive attitude on the part of the child to school and education in general. When one considers the formative nature of the child's early days in school it seems a great pity that the primary school teacher is not more carefully selected and given a higher status. Many children have been permanently turned against learning through being first exposed to a teacher who neither understands young children nor has a clear conception of the teacher's correct role at this stage.

A common complaint among school teachers is that they can cope with the children but not the parents and it is certainly true that the wrong attitude on the part of the parent can undo all the good brought about by an understanding teacher. We have already referred to the harmful effects on the children of parents who use them as instruments for bringing out their own unsatisfied longings. There is little doubt that some parents have already a preconceived idea of their child's future career before the child even enters school. It is a natural enough error for a parent to over-estimate his child's abilities but when the gulf between parental pride and the actual intelligence of the child becomes too wide the child is likely to be faced with demands which he cannot possibly meet. Equally harmful of course is the other extreme where the inherently bright child is held back in developing his ability by an inadequately stimulating home background. With the aid of understanding family support and the correct educational atmosphere the child will be allowed to develop his potentialities to their maximum limit.

Possibly we also tend to under-estimate the degree of adjustment which the child is called upon to make on first starting school. Even in the case of children who appear to accept this new life immediately without any concern, they often betray their true ambivalent feelings by their subsequent comments. Some time ago I was visiting the home of parents of a little boy who had recently started Sunday School. His parents were immensely pleased with this and were particularly happy that the little lad enjoyed these classes so much. Shortly after they had spoken, the boy himself returned from Sunday School and burst into the room declaring, 'Oh!

mummy, Sunday School was terribly good to-day, it was terribly exciting.' While the mother nodded in approval, father asked the little boy what made Sunday School so exciting to-day and the child replied, 'Oh! daddy, a little boy escaped!'

Psychological Disorders in Childhood

It is said that every age has its compensation but it would be equally true to say that every age has its own problems. In this section we will consider briefly a number of psychological problems which are associated with childhood.

The practice of classifying behavioural abnormalities into syndromes or disease entities, each distinguished by a set pattern of symptoms, is often difficult to apply reliably to adult disorders. In the case of psychological disorders in childhood, problems of classification are even more acute.

Many 'disturbed' children demonstrate *developmental* problems in that their behaviour is a problem only in so far as it does not accord with the chronological age of the child. Thus, enuresis, grossly uneven sleep rhythm, and egocentrically impulsive behaviour are all acceptably normal behaviours in infants and very young children. Such behaviours may only be regarded as maladjusted if they persist into or reappear in later childhood. In addition, whereas the behavioural patterns of adulthood are relatively enduring and consistent, those of the still developing child tend to be extremely labile and transient. The personality of the young child is still in the process of finding itself and many behaviours will appear fleetingly before a uniquely characteristic set of reactions is established. Much more so than the adult, the child's behaviour is being constantly influenced and shaped by external events and, in particular, by the reactions of others to the child's actions. If a new behaviour proves successful, as a means of either relieving tension or obtaining gratification and attention from others, the probability of its future reoccurrence will be increased. Should it continue to be so reinforced, it may eventually become part of the child's permanent personality. Conversely, if a new behaviour does not evoke such positive reactions from others, it will be more likely to dissipate and eventually to disappear from the child's repertoire of behaviours.

However, it would be a mistake to view the young child as a passive piece of clay whose final shape will be determined wholly by the actions of others in his interpersonal environment. Most mothers who have reared a large family of children will testify that no two children are alike, and they may further add that such individual differences are apparent from the earliest days of infancy. Studies of infantile behaviour support this view. In early infancy children show measureable differences in such functions as general activity level, regularity of hunger, sleep and excretion, adaptability to change and emotional responsiveness. Such individual differences seem unlikely to be caused by different methods of child rearing as they are apparent during the earliest stages of infancy, at a time when the environment has not had time to make much impact on the infant. The implication is that some facets of personality are constitutionally determined. Longitudinal studies have indicated that many of these personality differences show a remarkable consistency in continuing throughout the child's life. Thus, the infant who demonstrates an early readiness to adapt to environmental change later responds without stress to subsequent new experiences such as weaning, toilet training, starting school, etc. In assessing the many complex factors which determine our adult personality structure, we would do well to keep in mind that not all our virtues or our faults can be laid at the door of the long-suffering parents who reared us. The manner of child rearing adopted by the parents must in some measure be a reaction to the constitutionally predetermined mode of behaviour shown by each individual infant. The finished product which we call our personality is the result of a complex interplay between constitution and environment.

These comments are also pertinent to many of the psychological disorders of childhood.

Perhaps the most frequently met psychological upset during childhood is that of enuresis. It is the most important single factor accounting for the attendance of children at child guidance clinics, and a large number of untreated children continue bed-wetting well into late childhood or even into adulthood. Estimates vary but there would appear to be a proportion of around 10 per cent of enuretic children whose problem is primarily a physical abnormality directly inhibiting normal bladder control. Although such children constitute a relatively small minority of enuretic children, it would be a mistake to assume that the majority of bed-wetters are reflecting underlying emotional problems. Of course, this explanation is valid in some cases. For example, a child may react to the trauma of being displaced by the arrival of a new baby by reverting to an earlier phase of development. In wetting the bed, the child demonstrates his own need for attention and affection, which are now being lavished on the new arrival. Enuresis may again occur as a result of the anxiety aroused by separation, and many children react in this way when first coming into hospital. Children, in fact, react in many forms to emotionally disturbing situations and bed-wetting is undoubtedly one such reaction. If the underlying cause is of this type, one would expect the enuresis to clear up with the removal of the situation producing it and bed-wetting of this type is most often of a temporary nature. The habit may, however, be strengthened and the underlying emotional disturbance intensified by lack of understanding on the part of the adults responsible for handling the child. Direct punishment or the practice of attempting to shame the child out of his enuresis is seldom successful and usually only serves to worsen the situation. A simple appraisal of the possible situation to which the enuresis may be a reaction is more often likely to produce the most direct results. However, in the majority of cases, the aetiology appears to be somewhere between the two extremes of being purely physical or purely emotional. Studies indicate that most enuretic children fall into two discrete categories that are more directly related to the training regime per se than any other underlying causes. These categories consist of children who were trained too early and too rigidly and children who have received virtually no training. Treatment of the latter group presents few difficulties, merely taking the form of introducing the child to the toilet training which has hitherto been absent. Such children often come from homes where large families, general living conditions, and the lack of parental interest combine in leaving the child to rear himself. Treatment in the case of the other category, composed of children whose toilet habits break down after early training, is somewhat more difficult and prolonged. As we have already commented, most children spontaneously adapt themselves to toilet training at around the age of 15 months through imitation of parents and siblings. Although this represents the most desirable sequence, it involves a great deal of patience and work on the part of the mother and one can readily sympathize with mothers who prefer to establish some degree of toilet training at a much earlier age, although, as we have already commented, there can be no conscious control by the child during his first year. The real difficulty is that many adults who advocate early training do so out of an unhealthy attitude towards hygiene or, more specifically, an abnormally strong abhorrence of the child's excretory functions. The child's control over these functions is of such emotional importance to the mother that training is severely rigid and any lapse on the part of the child is treated as a major catastrophe. Apart from the anxiety this may raise in the child, the parental attitude may have the effect of emotionally over-weighing the whole toilet situation in the child's mind. In such a case, there is obviously more chance that the child will later react to emotional disturbance by a breakdown in his previously stable toilet habits.

As the majority of cases of enuresis are the product of faulty training, it is perhaps not surprising that the most effective forms of intervention involve a retraining approach. The most commonly used method employs pads inserted between the bed-sheets. As soon as the sleeping child begins to micturate, the dampness completes an electrical circuit, setting off a buzzer which wakes the child. The child is initially trained to rise and pass urine when wakened by the buzzer. Through a process of conditioning, the child eventually wakens to the stimulus of a full bladder and the apparatus can be dispensed with. This simple approach is so effective in the majority of cases that the manufacturers of the 'pad-buzzer' equipment often offer an unconditional return of the cost if results are not forthcoming after a fairly short period of use.

Although enuresis is a common symptom of maladjustment in childhood, it is obviously by no means the only one. We have already commented on the emotional immaturity typical of childhood, and many of the psychological disorders at this time are in fact an exaggeration of normal emotional responses. Temper tantrums, aggressiveness, and anxiety associated with various childhood fears are, for example, some of the most frequently found forms of emotional disturbances in children. The underlying disturbance may also be manifested in the form of anti-social behaviour such as habitual lying, stealing, and the whole gamut of delinquent behaviour. A final group of 'symptoms' which may result in the child appearing at a psychological clinic come under the heading of abnormal sexual behaviour. In general such disorders can only be defined as such in the eyes of worried parents who are not aware of the universal normality of such 'complaints' as masturbation and sexual curiosity in young children. This type of behaviour invariably results in a true personality disorder only after the child has incorporated an over-exaggerated sense of guilt from the reactions of his parents. It is worth pointing out here that many of the apparently pathological fears shown by disturbed children are simply patterns of behaviour learned from their parents. One often finds, for example, that some of the specific fears (e.g. fear of the dark, fear of blood, fear of animals, etc.) reported by young children have previously been apparent in the grandparents and beyond. We do not mean to imply that such fears are inherited, but rather that the child learns them through his contact and identification with his parents. Some years ago, in attending a children's clinic, I and my colleagues noticed a definite increase in the number of children whose main referral symptom was that of an acute fear that they would be attacked in bed at night by some sort of monster. This occurred at a time when there had been a series of murders in the town and it was not difficult to trace the derivation of the children's fear. Many mothers had in previous weeks been carefully locking their windows at night, fitting new locks to their doors and taking other precautions against the fears aroused by the fact that a dangerous man was at large in the community. The child's fear of attack in the night was only a representation of the fantasies aroused in the mind of the mother in this situation.

Depressive illnesses are much more common in later childhood then is commonly realized, although rarely found in younger children. At times the seriousness of the depression is made evident only in tragic retrospect by a suicidal act. A personality change in the older child or early adolescent involving loss of interest and energy, excessive fatigue, and feelings of being unwanted should always be viewed with caution.

One of the most severe forms of childhood disturbance is known as childhood autism. This condition often has been confused with childhood schizophrenia, a variant of the adult schizophrenic state, occurring infrequently in older children. However, more recent studies (Rutter and Lockyer, 1967; Kolvin *et al.*, 1971) have done much to establish that autism is a distinct form of childhood psychoses which runs a quite different course from childhood schizophrenia. The onset of autism is usually evident within the first few years of life and is characterized by gross speech disorder (to the point of complete muteness), ritualistic and compulsive behaviour and, above all, a profound impairment in the child's relationship with older people. It is this latter symptom of complete disinterest in interpersonal contact from which the term autism was originally derived. Opinions vary greatly as to the cause of this severe disorder, some arguments implicating pathological features in the parental–infant interaction, and others suggesting that the primary breakdown is due to organic malfunctioning in the central nervous system. Recent systematic research reports (e.g.

Kolvin *et al.*, 1971), reporting a higher incidence of pregnancy and delivery complications, abnormal EEGs, other neurological signs and the later emergence of epileptic seizures in autistic children would seem to support the view of an organic causality.

In contrast to autism, the other major psychosis of childhood, pre-adolescent or *childhood schizophrenia*, tends to have a later age of onset (after the age of 5 years and usually not before 8 years) and yields a clinical picture very similar to the adult form of the condition, which we shall be considering in a later chapter. Some cases (about 12 per cent) of childhood schizophrenia show a past family history of schizophrenia, thus indicating a genetic component. Evidence supporting an inherited factor in autism is rarely found.

Fortunately, these very malignant disorders of childhood are relatively uncommon. Psychoses in any form in childhood have an incidence of only 4.5 per 10,000. Childhood autism is found only in about 0.45 per 10,000 children.

A final category of childhood mental disorder of a different nature is that of mental deficiency. It need hardly be said that mental deficiency in the child is invariably a heavy blow to the parents and in fact many parents have great difficulty in accepting the condition and its irreversibility. Reactions of parents are varied. Although most learn to adjust themselves to the facts, others emotionally reject the mentally defective child, focusing their affections on the other normal members of the family. Other parents make a partial adjustment but, while their affection for the child remains unaffected, they torture themselves with feelings of guilt which are unfounded on fact. If the defect is a severe one, the child may require institutional care and the parents' guilt may be intensified by the separation. Many mentally defective children are, however, capable of assimilating varying degrees of training, and a surprising number are able to obtain work of a relatively simple and repetitive nature. Training schools which provide such facilities are too few, but those which exist do a magnificent job requiring endless patience and understanding. Steps are now being taken to provide more day hospitals where the mentally defective child may profit from the training without this involving complete separation from the parents. The majority of mental defectives are fortunately of the feeble-minded category (the highest grade of mental deficiency where the I.Q. is between 50 and 70 is referred to as feeble-mindedness to distinguish it from the lower grades of imbecility and idiocy) and quite capable of benefiting from suitably orientated education and of earning an independent living. Such higher grade defective children attend special day schools where the educational tempo is adjusted to their abilities. Obviously, the rather backward child will be much happier in such a setting than if he is left exposed to the unfair competition of the ordinary type of school. Unfortunately, one of the greatest drawbacks to adequate adjustment of parents and their mentally defective children is the social stigma and the social isolation so often imposed by the community. Other children can be cruel in their behaviour to the mentally defective child in their neighbourhood, but their sadism is merely an overt expression of the attitude of their parents. Finally, it is worthy of comment that numerous investigations have demonstrated that the child's mental level may be severely retarded by emotional disorder. Children who develop under the care of an overprotective mother, for example, who has a deep-seated neurotic need that her child remain dependent upon her may appear to be much lower intellectually than is the true case. In situations such as this, it has been shown that understanding psychological treatment of both mother and child can result in an apparent increase of intelligence to the extent of 20 I.Q. points.

To anyone who has studied closely psychological development in childhood, it soon becomes obvious that the familiar cliché of childhood being the happiest days of our lives is of very dubious validity. Although, on the surface, the everyday life of the young child may appear to be one of carefree irresponsibilities, we have seen that the child is being constantly called upon to make adjustments to changes, both within himself and in response to the demands made of him by others. Growing up is not an easy process and the child finds himself constantly bewildered and perplexed by a world to which he must eventually adapt himself.

At the same time, we must not fall into the opposite pitfall of overestimating the effects of childhood experiences on future personality development. It is too frequently assumed that the genesis of our adult personality, particularly its problems and conflicts, is entirely determined by childhood experience. In our studies of adult patients, we may trace their difficulties back to specific events (such as early separation from the mother) in childhood. From such retrospective studies we form a hypothesis that certain events in childhood are closely related to mental breakdown in adulthood. When, however, we attempt to use this apparent knowledge to make predictions regarding the future development of children who are being at present subjected to these same childhood experiences, we find that our system breaks down as the expected influence on later development does not take place. In recent years some research workers have begun to question this general assumption of the vital importance of childhood as setting a mould for later personality development. Reports on such investigations (e.g. Orlansky, 1949) tend to offer little support to the assumed direct link between, for example, certain child-rearing practices and the development of personality traits in later life. In examining the influence of early experiences on later personality development, one might conclude that, although some experiences might be acutely disturbing to the developing child, it is nevertheless dangerous to presume that such an effect will be long lasting and will distort subsequent development. Perhaps we have in the past tended to underrate the child's capacity for adjustment, forgetting that, although children are more impressionable than adults, they may at the same time be more resilient and adaptable. Perhaps we have tended to exaggerate the effects of environmental experience on personality development by underestimating the influence of constitutional differences.

The Child in Hospital

In this section we will finally consider some of the problems which arise when the child enters hospital. It is impossible to consider this question adequately until we have obtained some understanding of the psychological development of the child at various stages, which enables us to appreciate the practical problem of the child in hospital.

All forms of illness which result in hospitalization raise the problem of separation from the home. In recent years a considerable amount of work has been expended on endeavouring to assess the psychological effects on the child of this separation imposed by hospitalization. We have already referred to the work of Dr Bowlby whose conclusions have already been communicated directly to most nurses concerned with the treatment of children. Many readers will be familiar with the film *The Two Year Old goes to Hospital*, which provides a living record of the traumatic effect of separation from the mother at this stage of development. From what we have said already regarding the first year of life it will be evident that our interpretation of the effects of mother-child separation during this period must necessarily be different from the possible effects at a later age. It will be remembered that the child's capacity to conceive of, and form relations with, permanent objects in the environment appears to develop somewhere towards the end of the first year. In practice, this means that the child who is hospitalized before his world has become one of separate and identifiable individuals with a permanent existence would not be expected to show the same separation anxiety which characterizes the behaviour of the older child. Observations of children in hospital during this period confirm such a view and indicate that most infants settle down quite easily in hospital so long as the nursing care given is an adequate substitute for the mother in gratifying the infant's needs and demands. Difficulties might, however, arise if the infant were actually in hospital over the period when he first develops an awareness of permanent objects. One might expect, for example, in the case of an infant of six months being admitted to hospital for a lengthy period, that the first permanent relationship established would be between the child and the nurse who cares for him. In such circumstances the traumatic aspect of the situation as far as the child is concerned would actually occur when he had to leave hospital and adapt himself to establishing a new relationship with the mother. In such a case it might almost be more correct to speak of the anxiety aroused by the nurse-child separation.

In the case of the older child who has already established a permanent relationship with the mother, which is the basis of his security, separation by hospitalization must be a bewildering and highly traumatic experience. In such circumstances there is little wonder that the child reacts with overt manifestations of his anxiety in the form of crying, refusing to eat, disturbed sleep, and so forth. His anxiety may be temporarily alleviated by regular visits by his mother but, as most nurses are well aware, the inevitable aftermath of such visits is a renewal of anxiety and disturbed behaviour on the part of the child. Many people working in children's hospitals not unnaturally form the opinion that visiting is more a curse than a blessing and obviates the child settling down and adapting himself to the hospital routine. This is undoubtedly true as far as it affects the smooth running of the hospital, but as always, the main person to be considered is the patient. If the child has to be admitted to hospital and during the period of hospitalization be denied any contact with his parents one might expect him to feel that he had been thoroughly rejected. Regular visiting constitutes the only remaining link for the child with the security of his previous existence and, by denying him this small crumb of comfort, we may in fact make more permanent the break in his important relationship with his parents, particularly his mother. Many follow-up studies have indicated that children who feel rejected while in hospital tend to react in an emotionally disturbed manner when they finally return to their parents. Most children show some negative reactions on return home but, in the case of the child who has had little or no contact with his parents while in hospital, the reaction may be greatly exaggerated, causing not only a disturbance in the child but feelings of anxiety and guilt on the part of the parent. This raises the allied question of the effects upon parents of the hospitalization of their children. The mother-child separation is a reciprocal one and most mothers experience their own measure of anxiety on being separated from their child. This problem is often complicated by the mother's feeling of guilt stemming from the usually quite irrational fear that the child's illness is a reflection upon her care. Nurses will again be familiar with the manifestation of such feelings in the behaviour of parents during hospital visiting although they may not always recognize the source of the parents' annoying behaviour. Thus some parents will be over-fussy and critical of the care which is being given to their children, while others will react by an obvious display of their own anxiety and bewilderment making them difficult to handle and also disturbing the child. Such considerations have led some authorities to suggest that where possible the mother should enter hospital with the child and remain there during the course of his illness. While one cannot help but admire the idea behind such suggestions one must have grave doubts about their practicability. Apart from the merely physical problems of space and provision for the mothers in hospital it would only be in a considerably restricted number of cases that such an arrangement could be made. For example, a mother who had other children at home would find it extremely difficult and would gain little by allaying the separation anxiety of one child by creating the same anxiety in her other children. It would be highly undesirable to have children's wards where some mothers remain with the children while others could make an appearance only during the visiting hours. Perhaps a more realistic answer to the problem is for the nursing staff to have some understanding of the problem as it affects not only them but the child and the family and thus be able, by their understanding, to minimize the disturbances which arise when treating the child in hospital.

Although the effect of separation on the hospitalized child has been the subject of much study and debate there are, of course, other aspects of the situation to be considered. We have already commented on the young child's lack of true appreciation of death other than in terms of separation. This characteristic saves the child from the fear of death which is a chief source of anxiety among adult patients in hospital. However, this advantage is more than outweighed by the multitude of irrational fears which may be aroused by illness and hospitalization. I remember a child once telling me of her friend who had gone into hospital to undergo an operation. When I asked her if she had ever been in hospital, she replied: 'No, I'm a good girl!' Children, in fact, often associate illness requiring hospitalization as a form of punishment for their misdeeds and this fact in itself may make the child respond with fear to entering hospital for the first time. The unfamiliar surroundings, the uniforms, and the sight of equipment which makes the dentist's chair seem comfortable in comparison, all combine to enlarge the child's fears of what might be in store. Some children will react to the situation with a defensive muteness and negative unco-operative behaviour. Others will partially voice their fears by pestering the staff with questions. It is important for the nurse to realize that the child is not silent through sheer stubbornness nor will brief rational explanations satisfy his repeated inquiries. He seeks merely for someone to fill his mother's role by providing gentle comfort, reassurance, and sympathy in order to allay his anxiety. In a later chapter we will be discussing the 'personality defence mechanisms' which people adopt in times of stress. One of these mechanisms, 'regression,' refers to our tendency to return to an earlier and more primitive mode of behaviour when faced with a situation beyond our scope. The child commonly responds to hospitalization with a regressive reaction which may take the form of bedwetting, outbursts of temper, or any behaviour more appropriate to an earlier age level. Once again this type of disturbed behaviour indicates, not spitefulness calling for firm handling, but anxiety demanding patience and understanding.

It might be thought that an unnecessarily gloomy picture of the child in hospital has been painted here. Reactions will vary with age, with the illness, and with the individual. A normally neglected and lonely child may, for example, react with enthusiasm to the company of other patients and to the love and attention of the nursing staff. Some readers, who have worked in children's departments, may feel that they have learned little new in this section and that the problems we have mentioned have been made plain to them in their everyday work. If so, this is excellent, but it is only too easy in the hectic routine of hospital nursing to forget that the child presents special problems which are often related more to hospitalization than to his illness. An excellent and more detailed review of these problems is contained in a series of articles by H. R. Schaffer (1957) which is recommended to readers who wish to pursue the subject further.

Concluding Remarks

Let us finally attempt to summarize some of our impressions of this phase of personality development. The psychological study of the child is vital to our understanding of personality in general for there is little doubt that a great deal of the groundwork of our adult personality is laid down in those early years. We shall also see later that knowledge of early development is important in our attempts to understand mental breakdown in later life in so far as the primitive mental processes which govern the behaviour of the mentally ill have a striking correspondence with the normal mental processes of infancy and childhood. Psychological observation has allowed us some insight into the hitherto inaccessible world of the young infant whose main task during the first year is in emerging from the original adualistic fusion between self and environment and attaining a progressively clearer conception of the self as distinct from other objects. Throughout later childhood thinking is still egocentric and not fully adapted to reality. Perhaps the most important factor we learn from these studies is just this very fact of the wide differences between the thinking of the child and that of the adult. It is obvious that any attempt to understand or deal with children purely from the logical, reality orientated view of adulthood is bound to result in misunderstanding and failure. To understand the child we must be prepared to enter his world and the only possible key to it is our appreciation of the prelogical, magical nature of his thinking and feeling. It is only through the behaviour of the adults around him that the child gradually emerges from his inner world to become a socialized being adapted to reality. This process of adaptation may be delayed or made more difficult by the failure of the environment to provide a secure, stable, and encouraging background to development. The psychological emphasis on allowing the child to express himself and thus to develop his own individuality does not argue against a guiding discipline. Indeed, it is only through the impact of such rules of guidance that the child becomes a socialized being.

The many difficulties which make the observation and understanding of early development a challenge to our patience and ingenuity also make this field a fertile sowing ground for psychological hypothesis. Unfortunately, many of these hypotheses have come to be regarded as established facts widely adopted as such by people concerned with the practical business of child-rearing. One cannot help but feel that the uncritical acceptance of some unchecked psychological theories is perhaps of equal harm as the opposite attitude of overall denial of the importance of psychological data. The most vital gap in our knowledge concerns the permanency of childhood experience. One of the characteristics of the human personality is that it is constantly changing during the entire course of development. Childhood is commonly recognized as being a more plastic phase in that experiences at this time can mould the personality into specific and permanent patterns. In actual fact we have little psychological evidence to verify this general assumption. There is little doubt that certain childhood experiences may leave effects which persist into adult life. However, we as yet lack the knowledge to allow us to be anything but tentative in our conclusions as to which specific types of experience exert a permanent influence and we must accept an equal lack of certainty in attempting to predict what the future outcome of these experiences will be. Recent years have seen a growing awareness among psychologists of the need to establish the validity of their theories of child development and some writers (*e.g.*, Stevenson, 1957) have even questioned our assumption that childhood is the most malleable phase of human development.

It is important that the nurse, both in her role in treatment and in her capacity as a professional worker in the field of preventive medicine, be aware of both the scope and the limitation of present psychological knowledge of early development. She should also remember in her dealings with children and parents that no mother has yet borne or reared the average child which forms the criteria for many of our ideas governing the physical and natural development of the child. The conception of normal development based on the average allows us only guiding principles which, if too rigidly and emphatically applied, can result only in a distortion of the variability and lack of conformity in human behaviour.

QUESTIONS

1. To understand the child's behaviour we must appreciate the way in which he thinks. Describe some of the differences between the egocentric thinking of the child and the more logical thinking of the adult.

2. If asked to advise a parent, how would you summarize the most important family influences which affect the child's development, paying particular attention to such factors as habit, training, and discipline?

3. Describe some of the reactions you might expect from the young child in hospital. How would the nurse's understanding of these reactions assist her in her nursing of sick children?

2. Adolescence

By the time the child is twelve years his thinking is predominantly reality-orientated and relatively free from egocentricity. He has developed a wide range of skills and aptitudes which allow him to deal competently with most situations in his limited environment. He is by now well adapted, integrated and enjoys the security of an established social status within his own age group. By this age parents are beginning to relax and feel with relief that out of the earlier turmoil has emerged a reasonably stable adult in miniature. Suddenly, their well-earned tranquillity is shattered by a whole sequence of alterations in their child's behaviour. Integration and boyish confidence is replaced by disintegration, intense seld consciousness and the domestic scene is rent asunder by a series of emotional explosions. Adolescence has arrived!

Adolescence is essentially a period of physical, mental and social changes. The rate of growth curve shows a sudden marked spurt around adolescence which in boys is accompanied by a pronounced increase in strength and muscularity. Indeed, the muscular strength of the average boy tends to double itself within a two-year period during adolescence. The acceleration in growth occurs in girls around two years earlier but is accompanied by the same muscular changes. However, there is of course no such child as the 'average' adolescent, and there is a fairly wide scatter in the times when these changes occur in different youngsters. Thus two children may be of equal height at the age of 11 years and one outstrip the other by 4½ inches by the age of 14 years. In the subsequent three years the late maturer may then show an accelerated growth so that by the age of 17 years the two youngsters are again of equal height. Similar wide differences are found in breast development in girls, which may cause psychological problems both for the very early and very late maturer. The age at which sexual maturity is attained varies so widely that some children will have completed their sexual maturation before others of a similar age have even started.

The many physical changes which occur at this time cause the adolescent to be more aware of himself, more self-conscious in a literal sense. This new awareness of himself is intensified by the maturation of the secondary sexual characteristics, and reawakening of the long dormant sexual drive. How adequately youngsters learn to control and direct their sexual feelings partially depends upon the present and past attitudes of others, particularly their parents. Puberty also entails a new social adjustment in that popularity with the opposite sex is now an important symbol of social status.

The main mental change in adolescence is in the area of intellectual development. The young person of this age is equipped, not only with a new fund of physical energy, but also with a new fund of mental energy. In essence the adolescent becomes capable of a much more abstract mode of thinking and the capacity for new learning reaches its peak, slowly declining later in adulthood. For the first time he can deal with theories of an abstract nature and logically plan future projects. These aspects of intellectual development help to explain some typical features of adolescent behaviour. The new-found ability to reason in a wider context leads to endless speculations about abstract issues and new ideologies. The attitude to parents may be altered by the new capacity to question their reasoning and the realization that age does not necessarily bring wisdom. Finding that long-established sources of authority have feet of clay, the young person is likely to seek new authority figures, often nearer to his own age level. This accounts to some extent for the rebellious, non-conforming attitude of the adolescent who constantly debunks all sources of the no-longer infallible adult authority. Although this may be a trying period for the demoted parent, it is an essential and healthy part of development which aids the youngster in finding his own identity.

Even more confusing for the already bewildered parents is the fact that rejection by their adolescent children is seldom complete. Periods of rebellious hostility or indifference may be quickly followed by periods of dependence when the youngster again seeks for a short time the comfort and security of parental understanding and advice.

Adolescence is finally, and perhaps most importantly, a period of social change and adjustment. Although childhood and adulthood have their own problems they offer the individual a secure and clearly defined social role. The adolescent is asked to surrender the dependency of childhood without being offered the independency of adulthood. During this period of apprenticeship for manhood or womanhood the adolescent's social role is a vague, nebulous and often contradictory one. To some extent this long period of apprenriceship is imposed upon the young person by the society in which he lives. He may be criticized for being childish by the same adults who disparage and discourage his attempts to play a more mature role. It is not surprising that the adolescent inbetweens form their own social group or that their activities reflect their rootlessness and their insecure state of mind. In some less advanced societies adolescence does not exist as a distinct stage of human development. In such societies the child is accepted as such until he reaches a certain age. At this point he is fully accepted as a responsible adult member of his social group and assigned a clearly defined role to play. It is not surprising that many of the emotional and behavioural problems which appear to us as being a natural part of adolescence are much less evident in such societies.

What are the effects of such changes on the adolescent personality? Their main effect is probably summed up in one word—uncertainty. The adolescent suffers from a basic lack of direction. His own emotions are confused and ambivalent. He senses his own mental power but at the same time lacks the inner confidence to translate his beliefs into a definite course of action. His delight in shocking his parents' adult composure is matched by the feelings of guilt which his own behaviour invokes. Fantasies and day-dreams are an easy substitute for action and in such imaginative reveries all problems are solved. In these he is sophisticated, sexually dominant, respected by others and decisive in action. Later, if he is to reach a more mature level of development, he must come to some sort of compromise between his inner desires and outward achievements. Out of this maelstrom of conflicting feelings and ideas the adolescent must find a new individual identity. He must find for himself what sort of person he is, where he is going in life and what are his personal limitations and potentialities. Some psychologists have called the adolescent period a crisis of identity, to stress the crucial process of social and personal readjustment involved.

Psychological Disorders in Adolescence

The main difficulty in discussing mental health in adolescence is in differentiating between the true psychological disorder or neurosis and the reactions to adolescence itself. In essence every neurotic reaction represents a faulty adjustment to the social environment. The failure of the individual to make a satisfactory adjustment may occur when the environment makes impossible demands on the individual. The failure may also have an 'internal' cause in that the individual lacks the maturity and stability to face his social environment. In most cases the cause of neurotic disorder lies somewhere between these two extremes involving both the individual's approach to his environment and the effects of the environment upon him.

The adolescent is often a rather insecure, anxious person bewildered by the many changes which are taking place over the adolescent period. In response to this situation many adolescents behave in ways which are regarded by the more mature adult as being abnormal. Certainly, the behaviour of many young people, judged in the context of our more stable and secure adult existence, would appear to deviate from normal standards. When this behaviour is understood, however, in the background of the period of adolescent development, we can see that much of the young person's apparently odd behaviour is an only too normal reaction to an abnormal situation. The sources of disturbance in adolescence may be manifold. Conflict with parents, vocational difficulties, overconcern with religious and philosophical issues, sexual problems, and in fact any of the trials and tribulations of growing up, may result in subjective feelings of anxiety and insecurity. It is only too easy for the adult observer to be condescending about the adolescent's frame of mind, regarding him as a 'crazy mixed up kid,' who will some day look back on this period with amusement. We tend to forget that much of the young person's concern and despair over the world in which he finds himself growing up is a genuine and spontaneous feeling with a great deal of positive value which may be constructively harnessed. While the adolescent's reactions to situations may be exaggerated and dominated by his emotions rather than by logic they are nevertheless often preferable to the resigned apathy and disinterestedness of the more 'mature' adult who attains stability and peace of mind only at the expense of his spontaneity and his social conscience.

The most common symptom of mental disorder in adolescence is that of anxiety in one form or another. Anxiety is, of course, a normal reaction to situations which threaten the individual, and people may be extremely anxious without being in any way neurotic. For the young soldier in wartime to be anxious about his own survival is only too normal and is in fact a healthy reaction which may aid him to survive. Neurotic anxiety, on the other hand, is indicated when there is an apparent lack of connection between the provoking experiences and the emotional reaction of the individual. At times the individual may, in fact, experience intense crippling anxiety without having any idea of its source. When the anxiety is 'free-floating,' in that it is not attached to any specific situation, the individual may be suffering from what is perhaps the most common neurotic reaction, not only of adolescence but also of adult life, the so-called *Anxiety State*. In this condition the person is haunted by devastating anxiety which fills him with a constant sense of apprehension and uneasiness. Having no awareness of the source of his fear he is unable to guard himself against it or to deal with it in a constructive way. The patient's inner anxiety may vary widely between a mild uneasiness to an acute *panic reaction*. In this latter state he may become acutely disturbed and be convinced that something dreadful is about to happen to him, that he may die or go out of his mind. As time goes on the patient becomes chronically anxious, feeling tense, restless, and showing a great deal of irritability in his relations with others. Intense anxiety is at times accompanied by the very terrifying experience that psychiatrists have termed *depersonalization*. In this state the person loses the sense of familiarity of his own body, feels he is losing his own identity and that he is cut off from the rest of the environment. Depersonalization may be accompanied by the allied experience of *derealization* where the individuals find that objects and persons outside of him seem strange and no longer familiar. These feelings of unreality are perhaps the most disturbing of all the alterations of experience which occur in anxiety states. Although transient, the patient may become convinced that he is losing contact with reality, and that he is becoming insane. Apart from these subjective mental symptoms, the patients suffering from this type of neurotic condition are likely to complain of a number of bodily symptoms. A rapid pulse with palpitations and disturbing sensations around the heart are common. The patient's anxiety may affect his breathing, and his efforts to compensate for this by breathing more deeply may give rise to feelings of giddiness. His digestive system is likely to be affected so that he is put off his food by constant feelings of nausea and even actual vomiting. He may also complain of weakness of the bladder and diarrhoea. His anxious state may be visible to others in spasmodic trembling of his limbs or in obvious signs of tension in his face. In acute panic attacks the patient may actually lose consciousness although the form of such fainting attacks are quite distinct from that seen in epileptic patients. The various physical symptoms which are typical of this type of neurotic reaction are likely to exert a further effect in causing the patient to become fearful about his physical state of health. He may feel that he is suffering from a heart condition or that the disturbances in his digestive system indicate a malignant disease such as cancer. Many patients who feel that they are going out of their mind become convinced that they are suffering from a brain tumour. Not unnaturally this type of reaction to the physical changes increases the patient's anxiety, so setting up a vicious circle of cause and effect to produce a chronic anxiety state. Reassurance that the condition, although disturbing, is not as serious as it may seem and certainly not fatal, may help in temporarily easing the patient's inner anxieties and the prescription of an appropriate sedative may dampen down the severity of his acute attacks. If it is possible to help the patient to achieve insight into the root cause of his neurotic reaction, the anxiety attacks may clear up, although it is likely that the patient will remain an overanxious type of person. The vast majority of young people who suffer from anxiety states respond fairly well to treatment.

The basic neurotic anxiety may, however, become focused on some particular situations and in this form the neurotic reaction would be termed a *Phobic State*. The patient may complain of a fear of traffic, of enclosed spaces, of travelling, or being alone, and, in fact, of any type or number of specific situations. Again, it is worthy of note that such phobias may differ from normal fears only by the lack of contiguity between the fear and the object which arouses it. A fear of snakes or wild animals would be regarded as normal in that the danger is a real one. In a similar fashion, a certain degree of fear reaction to heights may protect the individual from possible harm. The neurotic phobia is distinguished by the irrational nature of the fear, which is aroused by situations, not in themselves harmful to the individual. The crippling effect of the phobia will, of course, vary with the situation of the individual and the degree to which the object of the phobia figures in the person's everyday life. Thus, for example, a phobia directed at traffic would mean something quite different to the office worker living in town, as compared with a farm worker living in a rural district.

In other cases the anxiety may find a somatic outlet, the symptoms taking the form of fears in connection with bodily illness. Here the patient would be described as suffering from a *Hypochondriacal State* where he is constantly preoccupied with the subject of illness. He may haunt his doctor's consulting room with complaints of digestive disorder, symptoms of heart disease, cancer, and in fact, symptoms of any physical illness. Often a patient's hypochondriacal behaviour might at least attain the temporary object of achieving affectionate solicitude from others. It may also have the secondary effect of enabling the patient to manipulate and dominate others around him whose continual presence is important for the patient's security. Thus, the behaviour of a whole household may be organized around the hypochondriacal illnesses of one member of the family. In such cases the patient's fears may be alleviated by examination and medical reassurance but, unless the basic cause of the anxiety is unearthed, the patient is more likely to develop new hypochondriacal fears in the future. Where the anxiety is converted into a specific physical channel, resulting in the patient being physically disabled in some way, the psychiatrist would describe the disorder as a *Conversion Hysteria*. Some of the reactions to acute stress experienced by members of the Forces in war-time are typical illustrations of traumatic conversion reactions. The front-line soldier who is torn between his desire to protect himself by running away on the one hand, and his sense of duty on the other, may solve his conflict by becoming paralysed in the limbs. He is then literally in a position where he is unable to go on to fight and equally unable to turn back and run. At times it is extremely difficult to differentiate between symptoms of conversion hysteria and a physical disability with an underlying organic cause, and the differential diagnosis requires expert medical assessment. There seems no doubt that many of the sudden and miraculous recoveries from a disabling illness indicate that the disablement was in the nature of a conversion symptom. Again there are many examples of temporary conversion symptoms which are still within the bounds of normal rather than abnormal behaviour. The dramatic loss of speech, constituting a temporary aphonia, which occurs in cases of stage fright, is a typical example here and one might also cite at least some of the cases occurring in the well-known phenomenon of 'night-nurse's paralysis.' One must be careful in speaking of hysteria to distinguish between conversion hysteria as here described and the *hysterical personality*. Hysterical personality is a term which refers, not to a form of psychiatric illness, but to a recognizable personality type. We use this term to describe the sort of person who is essentially egocentric, immature, and over-dependent in his relations with others. When faced with difficult decisions he tends to retreat into fantasies rather than face up to reality as it is. He is subject to emotional outbursts of a rather theatrical nature, his feelings being intense but superficial and transient. In his dealings with others he is excessively sentimental, insincere, and is capable of deceiving himself as often as he deceives others. The hysterical personality is essentially a play actor who has no real control over the parts he plays. It was at one time thought that individuals with an hysterical personality were more predisposed to develop symptoms of conversion hysteria in the case of a nervous breakdown. However, studies (e.g. Chodoff and Lyons, 1958) of the premorbid personality of patients suffering from conversion hysteria indicate that there is no direct causal link between this illness and the hysterical personality. In other words, conversion hysteria is not more likely to develop in people of an hysterical personality as compared with others of an entirely different personality make-up.

Other patients suffering from neurotic illnesses complain less of anxiety and bodily discomfort than of abnormally persistent ideas and impulses. They find themselves haunted by thoughts which are repetitive and compulsive in the sense that they are unable to control their emergence into consciousness. At times the recurring theme or idea may be trivial in nature, but often it takes the form of something which greatly distresses the individual and is completely foreign to his usual thinking. The intruding factor may take the form, not of an obsessional thought, but of a compulsive urge to behave in ways alien to the person's normal nature. Thus the patient may be afraid that he will be compelled to harm someone dear to him, the patient feeling himself compelled to indulge in a variety of useless and time-wasting rituals. He may, for example, feel compelled to repeatedly wash his hands, or to continually arrange objects around him in certain fixed and meaningless patterns. The patient whose symptoms take this form may be said to be in an *Obsessional-Compulsive* neurotic state. Such factors of course again arise in normal behaviour and most people have, from time to time, been affected temporarily by obsessional ideas or behaviour which are strangely compulsive. Many of us, after retiring to bed, have experienced the urge to recheck if the gas or electricity has been turned off although we know in our minds this has already been done. An acquaintance of mine whose behaviour is otherwise completely normal and controlled found himself compelled to jump up and touch the branches of a specific tree on his way to work each day. When he tried to resist this meaningless impulse he found himself strangely uneasy and anxious for the rest of the day. Some people are distinctly obsessional in their general personality make-up. We might describe the obsessional personality as one who is abnormally rigid and inflexible in his behaviour, and who encloses his personal life within a strict routine, defending himself against the unexpected which he always finds disturbing. Such people are likely to be fussy, meticulous, and pedantic in their everyday behaviour, continually making demands both of themselves and of others. There does seem to be sufficient evidence to indicate a direct link between previous personality make-up and obsessional neurosis. Studies of the premorbid personality of these patients indicate that they have always shown strong obsessional traits, this being often evident from early childhood. Many people suffering from a variety of neurotic conditions show, of course, minor obsessional traits in their symptoms. The true obsessional neurotic is, however, not difficult to diagnose in that the obsessional and compulsive elements in his behaviour are predominant. An important point of diagnostic significance in evaluating obsessional symptoms is that, in true obsessional neurosis, the patient is well aware of the irrational and useless nature of his compulsions and tries, although unsuccessfully, to resist them. Some schizophrenic patients in the early stages of their illness also show strong obsessional symptoms in their behaviour but these patients tend to accept, rather than resist, their obsessional tendencies. The apparently obsessional patient who later becomes clearly schizophrenic is more likely to see his obsessional and compulsive symptoms as having some sort of mysterious significance for him. Thus, one such patient who had a compulsive need to add numbers in his head felt that these numbers constituted a coded message from outer space. The classical obsessional neurosis is a comparatively rare condition and few psychiatrists see more than a very small number of these patients in a lifetime of practice.

It is often said that anxiety is the main reaction to stress during the first half of life while depression is a more typical reaction in the latter half of life. While this is in general true the *Neurotic Depression* reaction is also found quite commonly in elderly people. As in the case of anxiety reactions depressive feelings are, of course, part of everyday reactions to normal life and depression takes the form of a neurotic disorder only when the depressive feelings are so pronounced and long lasting as to disturb radically the individual's way of life. It would appear that some people are temperamentally predisposed to react to stress by becoming depressed and there is some evidence that women are more vulnerable to this form of reaction than men. The female reader will no doubt comment that women have more to become depressed about. Adolescents are characteristically unstable in their moods and may traverse the whole range of feeling from depression to elation in a very short space of time. Some young people do, however, react very strongly to the frustrations and disappointments which are a necessary consequence of this stage of life. Shyness and difficulty in finding one's place in the social group, unhappy love affairs, failure in examinations and other such minor catastrophes may be greatly magnified in the impressionable mind of the adolescent boy or girl and result in a moderate or severe depressive reaction. The frustrations of adolescence are, of course, not uniformly distributed and some young people collapse under an overload of environmental difficulties. In such cases the individual becomes excessively unhappy about the present and grossly pessimistic with regard to the future. As one intelligent adolescent girl remarked to the author: 'a black cloud seems to have settled over my life and I can't seem to see past it.' The depressed patient is haunted also by a strong sense of guilt which causes him to be preoccupied with minor misdeeds and to see himself as an unworthy person who does not deserve to be accepted or loved by others. He loses interest in the everyday events which formerly took up his attention and spends most of his time in solitary brooding. His state of mind may become obvious to his family and others by his disturbed sleep, poor appetite and his melancholy demeanour in general.

Treatment for the neurotic conditions which we have briefly described varies greatly with the severity of the illness. We have already implied that it is impossible to draw any clear-cut line which separates neurotic from normal behaviour. The neurotic patient is usually concerned with problems with which we are all familiar in our own lives and, as we have seen, his actual symptoms may be often understood as exaggerations of our own reactions to stress. In the case of a mild neurotic illness the opportunity for the patient to talk over his difficulties with an understanding doctor may indeed be all that is required. Many patients are vastly relieved merely by the knowledge that their symptoms are by no means unique, that they are not alarming and that they do not signify that the patient is going out of his mind. Many neurotic illnesses may be treated by the patient's own doctor or at an out-patient clinic by a mixture of reassurance and suitable sedation to dampen down the anxiety. Where the neurosis is most severe a course psychotherapy may be advisable under a psychiatrist suitably qualified to undertake this form of treatment. Psychotherapy takes a number of different forms, which are beyond the scope of this book to examine in detail. In general, however, all forms of psychotherapy have the common object of aiding the patient to work through his difficulties and attain some degree of insight into the source of his neurotic conflict. In the case of a phobic state, for example, the patient's symptoms may be alleviated by his achieving insight into the fact this his fears have been displaced from their true source which has hitherto been inaccessible to his own awareness. In successful treatment of this kind the patient might not only achieve alleviation of his immediate symptoms but also enough insight to allow him to perceive new patterns in his own behaviour which will give him a greater measure of control over himself in the future. Fortunately most neurotic disorders, particularly when they occur in young people, are transient and responsive to treatment. The majority of illnesses of this type would, in fact, probably improve and eventually clear up with the passage of time and the alleviation of the provoking factors in the environment. In some cases, however, the individual remains throughout life chronically anxious and neurotically vulnerable to any stressful situations. Some people, in fact, without ever having had a nervous breakdown as such, remain adolescents for most of their life, in that they never attain the degree of emotional maturity which denotes the attainment of a stable adult adjustment. We describe such people in everyday speech as 'childish' in their behaviour indicating their emotional immaturity and general inadequacy which prevents them adopting an adult role.

Another form of psychological reaction in adolescence is that of extreme *shyness and withdrawal* from social contacts. Many young people, particularly young girls, attend psychiatric outpatient departments with complaints of lack of confidence and inability to mix socially. Obviously we cannot all be the 'life and soul of the party,' nor would we all wish to be, but some degree of self-confidence and social ease is necessary for a happy and normal life. The insight and understanding of the doctor can often help the young person to be more at ease with his or herself and to be less vulnerable and sensitive to the slings and arrows of social demands. If the ultra-sensitive young person suffers too many rebuffs in his interactions with other people the result may be a progressive withdrawal from others with a corresponding tendency to day-dreaming and a diminution of interest in the real world. Some adolescents do indeed retire within themselves in this way, becoming more and more preoccupied with mystical and philosophical ideas at the expense of their interest in the more practical events which make up everyday life. When this withdrawal from objective reality and social contact becomes excessively pronounced and pervades all areas of the personality we may then have cause for concern that the change in behaviour represents the early symptoms of one of the most serious forms of mental illness, *schizophrenia*. This term does literally mean 'split-mind' but does not refer to the popular misconception of a person who lives a double life in the Jekyll and Hyde tradition. The split or 'schism' in this case is between the individual and reality for the illness results in a loss of contact with reality or, more precisely, a progressive diminution in the patient's capacity to differentiate between his own subjective internal world and the objective world outside him.

The earliest symptoms of schizophrenia may be very difficult to detect and the patient has himself great difficulty in expressing them in words. As some forms of the disease develop slowly and insidiously over a period of years, the illness may be well advanced before the patient first seeks treatment. Among the earliest reported symptoms are such as complaints of difficulty in concentrating, a flattening of affect so that the patient feels dull and uninterested, and a gradual withdrawal from social life. The clinical picture in the early stage may in fact be difficult to distinguish from that of a mild depressive state. In some forms of schizophrenia the illness develops much more suddenly and the first symptoms here are likely to be more acute and bizarre. The patient may experience severe feelings of unreality and feel that his own body is visibly changing. He has great difficulty in expressing his thoughts and may himself declare that his thinking is mixed up. The world around him seems itself altered and he is liable to read strange meaning and significance into trivial everyday events. The patient may soon feel that his thoughts are not only confused but that they are not his own and from this he may soon become obviously hallucinated, regarding his own thoughts as voices in his head which are influencing his behaviour. As the schizophrenic illness progresses the patient becomes more obviously disordered in his thinking which is vague, woolly, and difficult to follow. The meanings of words become altered for the schizophrenic in that he invests them with personal significance. Thus if passing neighbours happen to greet him with a customary 'good morning,' he may feel that they are really asking him if he has been good this morning and that this infers that they have some secret knowledge of his personal life. In the most malignant forms of the illness this disorder of thinking becomes progressively more severe until the patient appears to have lost all control of the direction of his thoughts. In the latter stages the disruption of the normal thinking process becomes so pronounced that the patient may be unable to communicate to others in a meaningful manner. Although this gradual deterioration in the thinking process is perhaps the most typical feature of a schizophrenic condition, there is also a noticeable change in the emotional life of the patient. Most frequently the patient shows an impoverishment of affect and his responses to emotionally arousing situations are likely to be completely apathetic. Thus he shows no interest or enthusiasm in former sources of enjoyment and loses any feelings of affection he once held towards others near to him. In some cases the emotional state is not so much one of apathy but of emotional responses which are inappropriate to the situation. Thus he may respond with laughter in a serious situation, or smile happily in situations which would normally have moved him to tears. The alterations in the patient's thinking and in his emotional life cause him to become more and more preoccupied with his own changing inner world and to progressively withdraw from all social contact. He is likely to lose interest in his appearance and to show a marked deterioration in social habits. Such contact as does remain with the outside world will be misperceived, and out of the patient's distorted view of his environment may arise bizarre hallucinations and delusions. The most common form of hallucinatory activity in schizophrenia is that of hearing voices, this appearing to develop from the patient's earlier inability to control his thoughts, which now seem alien to him. His sense of alienation may be completed by his growing conviction that other people are talking about him, acting against him, and interfering with his life. He may feel, for example, that people can read his thoughts or that they can project their own thoughts into his mind. His inability to control his own thoughts, feelings, and behaviour may cause him to believe that he is under the control of others who have hypnotized him or have some strange power over him. Although *paranoid delusions* of this type are quite common among the secondary symptoms of schizophrenia, they can in some cases constitute the patient's main or primary symptoms. Most psychiatrists now regard patients who show few or none of the primary symptoms of schizophrenia, particularly that of thought disorder, as being so different in their symptomatology and in the subsequent development of their illness as to constitute a separate psychotic illness, that of a *paranoid psychosis*. The onset of a paranoid psychosis usually occurs at a later age and the subsequent development of the illness is quite different from that of schizophrenia itself. The main symptoms are of a markedly suspicious attitude to others and a growing conviction in the patient's mind that all his misfortunes are caused by others who are united in some sort of plot against him. Sometimes the paranoid feelings reported are quite bizarre, as illustrated by the patient who became convinced that the Electricity Board was plotting against him by sending electrical charges through his television set, his water taps, and through the walls. As already stated, these patients do not show the same type of obvious thought disorder as that which is apparent in schizophrenic patients, and in speaking to them they may appear quite normal until the subject of their paranoid delusional system is touched upon. There is some evidence to suggest that the development of a paranoid illness may be more influenced by environmental circumstances than is the case with other psychotic conditions. There is, for example, an unusually high incidence of deafness among paranoid patients and these symptoms are not uncommon in elderly people who live in social isolation from other people.

These types of psychotic illnesses which we have been describing are obviously quite radically different from the neurotic disorders discussed earlier. The difference between these two categories of mental disorder has been described as follows: 'A psychotic lives, in so far as he is a psychotic, in a world of fantasy; a neurotic lives in the real world; his difficulties are greater by far for him than they are for normal people, but they are the same difficulties which all of us have. The difficulties of the psychotic arise from the fact that he is living in quite another world, in which one is not subject to the ordinary physical laws' (Ross, 1923). The other main type of psychotic illness is that of *Affective* psychosis. Here the disorder is fundamentally an emotional one in that the patient's mood may vary from the depths of depression to the heights of manic elation. This form of mental illness will be discussed in more detail in the later section dealing with adulthood. The prognosis and eventual outcome in the case of psychotic illnesses is obviously less favourable than in the case of a neurotic disorder. However, modern advances in the field of psychiatry have yielded methods of treatment which are proving fairly effective ways of coping even with these very disturbing illnesses. Psychiatrists are at present collaborating with scientists in other fields such as biochemistry and neurophysiology and their combined efforts are gradually giving us a greater understanding of the pathological mechanisms which result in a psychotic breakdown. The outlook here, then, is a great improvement from that which existed twenty years ago, although we are still far from understanding the basic causes of these conditions.

A final group of psychiatric disorders found in adolescence might be covered by the general term of *anti-social behaviour*. Most young people are anti-social to some extent in so far as they are rebels against the existing order of society, and such non-conformity is both a normal and healthy reaction. However, the occurrence of extreme rebellion in the form of juvenile delinquency creates a genuine and difficult social problem which causes much concern in the present day. Obviously it would be unrealistic to seek to find any one cause of such a complex reaction as delinquent behaviour. An unsatisfactory and insecure home life, a lack of positive moral values, the loosening of family and group ties, the social approval of easily accomplished material gain, the decline in religious faith, boredom, international unrest, and even the often exaggerated effects of television, films, and the 'horror-comic,' have all been seen as stimulating aggressive anti-social behaviour in easily influenced adolescents. Each of these arguments has some validity but we must judge every case of delinquency on its individual merits rather than attempt to apply any glib general formula. Some delinquent youths would possibly have benefited from a more socializing form of parental discipline while others have obviously reacted to over-severe and restrictive discipline. One might indeed argue that there are as many reasons for delinquent behaviour as there are delinquents. It may be useful, however, to consider delinquent behaviour as falling under three main categories. Under the first category we might place the transient types of mild delinquent behaviour which can occur as part of the customary pattern of rebellion shown by many adolescents. The young people in this category whose actions bring them before the court are usually first offenders, whose delinquency takes a mild form and who later settle down and become reasonably well-adjusted citizens. In the second category of delinquency we might place those individuals whose delinquency is a symptom of an underlying emotional disturbance. Many of these young people come from homes in which the parents have shown little interest in their child's welfare or, in some cases, from homes which have been greatly disturbed by parental disharmony. This leaves us with the third and largest sector of delinquent behaviour, composed of children whose social background conditions them towards anti-social behaviour. Studies of the social background of these 'sub-cultural' delinquents reveal an unusually high incidence of criminal behaviour in other members of the family, particularly among their fathers. The child's delinquency here may simply be due to the usual process of identification by which boys imitate and emulate their father's role. Delinquents in this category often belong to a cultural background that is at variance with the standards of behaviour characteristic of society as a whole. If we judge a delinquent youth by our own standard, he may be guilty of highly abnormal behaviour, which is nevertheless 'normal' in the sense of being well adjusted to the standards of the social group to which he belongs. This wide gulf in the standards of behaviour between different social groups is one of the greatest barriers to adequate communication and understanding between those who study and seek to eradicate delinquent behaviour and those who commit it. One of the best illustrations of the delinquent's point of view and of the barrier between him and those who would seek to 'improve' his standards of conduct is given in Sillitoe's powerful short story *The Loneliness of the Long Distance Runner* (1959). This fictional insight into the attitude of a young delinquent leaves us with a strong awareness of the enormous difficulties in handling this type of social problem. One can easily see that, unless we are able to bring about some basic change in the attitudes shown by such young people, they are most likely to develop into habitual criminals continually at war with society. Perhaps one of the clearest expositions of the basic standards of the habitual criminal has been given, not in a psychological textbook, but in the frank autobiographical account of an intelligent but confirmed criminal, appropriately entitled *The Courage of His Convictions* (1962). We can recognize in this true account the young delinquent in Sillitoe's story twenty years later and one is again appalled by the enormity of the problem facing those who seek to modify such deeply ingrained attitudes towards the rest of society. Finally, in our tendency to condemn out of hand the juvenile offender, we might perhaps first pause to remember that youth always tends in its behaviour to reflect in some measure the values of adult society. It is possible that the moral values in the world around us today are not wholly conducive to develop in many adolescents a sense of communal responsibility founded upon mutual respect and trust.

Apart from the normal delinquent, if one can be allowed such an expression, psychiatry is also faced with the smaller but important group of delinquents who at times have been described by the term *moral defective*. We have seen earlier in our discussion of childhood that the average child begins to develop a true moral sense somewhere around the age of 7 years. Normally this gradually develops as the child grows older so that he enters adolescence equipped with what we might call a social conscience. If for some reason the child is unable to attain this new level of development his moral sense will continue to operate at the rudimentary level of the younger child who has not yet internalized a set of moral standards. He may continue to develop normally in other ways and his intellectual ability, as measured, on a standard intelligence test, may be within normal limits or even be above average. His deficiency then is not an intellectual one as such, as in the case of a mental defective, but an impairment of judgment based upon the absence of a social conscience or a sense of moral values. Such people can be categorized under the term *Psychopath* which also describes the group of anti-social individuals, who throughout their life have been unable to conform to the moral and ethical demands of society. Such individuals are usually well aware of the deviant nature of their own behaviour and may repeatedly express themselves as being contrite and about to reform their habitual anti-social life patterns. However, their apparent insight is superficial and lacking in any real emotional depth. As one team of investigators puts it—'the psychopath knows the words but not the music' (Johns and Quay, 1962). Research tends to support the observation that psychopathic individuals tend to have unusually low levels of anxiety and that they fail to develop the normal fear responses to punishments which act as an internal deterrent to others. The behaviour of a proportion of this group tends also to be characterized by sudden and explosive outbursts of rage and aggressive behaviour. There is some evidence, which is not yet conclusive, that the brain rhythms of such people show an abnormality which indicates that their disturbance is basically similar to epilepsy. Although they may never show the typical attack, with convulsion and loss of consciousness, their outbursts of uncontrollable aggression may be due to the same cause, a minor brainstorm. The larger proportion of this diagnostic group are not, however, prone to such aggressive outbursts and their behaviour is characterized more by their immaturity and inadequacy in social situations. In some, this immaturity is reflected in their EEG activity which contains an unusually high proportion of the slow brain rhythms normally associated with young children. It has been suggested that some such people suffer from a delay in the maturation of the cortical centres which normally control and inhibit impulsive behaviour. Some support for this hypothesis is available from observations (Robins, 1966) that psychopathic behaviour decreases with age in adulthood, with a pronounced normalizing of behaviour often occurring between the thirtieth and fortieth years of life.

Some psychiatrists feel uneasy about the position of the so-called moral defective in that, while it is relatively simple to assess a person's intellectual level, it is a much more difficult question when we are asked to assess a person's level of moral judgment. It is also undoubtedly true that a mental deficiency institution is not the ideal place for a young person who is morally unsound, but intellectually normal. Indeed this whole subject of the treatment of the anti-social individual, whether he be termed a moral defective, psychopath or emotionally immature person, is a very pertinent one at the present moment. Some authorities who have examined the position, such as Barbara Wootton (1959), suggest that this category is outwith the boundary of medical and psychiatric treatment and that the problem is a social one which must be tackled along different lines. One of the main difficulties here, is that, while the diagnosis of, let us say, schizophrenia although complex, is obviously a psychiatric issue involving a fairly objective medical judgment, the diagnosis of moral deficiency or psychopathy infers a value judgment on human behaviour which some would argue the psychiatrist is not necessarily qualified to make. Many psychiatrists share this opinion, but at the present moment there exists no other agency which can deal with the referral and subsequent treatment of the moral offender.

The Adolescent as a Patient

It need hardly be said once again that, as in the case of all individuals, adolescents will react to illness in a variety of ways depending both on the illness itself and the personality of the patient. There are, however, certain aspects of illness and hospitalization which might be expected to affect the adolescent somewhat differently from patients in other age groups.

Perhaps one of the most obvious problems arises from the adolescent's increased awareness of his or her body which is a reaction to the physical changes which take place during puberty. During this period of physical change the young person, often abnormally shy and modest, may find the lack of privacy in hospital a little upsetting. I remember speaking to one adolescent boy who had found that the most trying experience of his daily life in hospital had been having to be bathed by a nurse. His embarrassment was made less acute than it might have been by the obviously objective and matter-of-fact attitude of his nurse, but one might imagine that if the nurse concerned had herself been an inexperienced adolescent the situation might have been most disturbing for the patient. The impressionable and over-emotional young person may again react in an exaggerated fashion not only to his or her own illness, but to the illnesses of other patients in the ward. Obviously it would be most desirable that the adolescent patient be surrounded, if possible, with other patients of his own age group. One might imagine that a young person who found himself in a bed next to an elderly patient who was seriously ill could be seriously disturbed and upset. Most young people are, in fact, possibly more sensitive to the suffering of others than they are to their own suffering. I have heard nurses comment that young people appear to be able to stand a remarkable amount of pain and discomfort without the complaints one might expect from many adult patients while they are, at the same time, over-sensitive to the pain and discomfort of other patients. One might expect, in fact, that in many ways the adolescent would be an ideal patient. Their illness represents a concrete problem to them which they can face with courage and a healthy determination to overcome it and get well as soon as possible. They are usually physically very resilient and are up and about at the earliest opportunity. A more likely nursing problem, in fact, is the indirect one of helping the adolescent patients to occupy themselves during this period of enforced immobility which cuts off the usual outlets for their energy. The enforced physical idleness and lack of activity during hospitalization may have the effect of turning the young person's attention inward towards himself. We have already noted that the adolescent has a vivid phantasy life and that there is usually a tendency towards day-dreaming. It is perhaps not always healthy to allow the adolescent's imagination to have a full rein without the corrective experiences of reality. The more, then, that one can keep the adolescent patient's interest and attention occupied in the world around him, either by participating as much as possible in the life of the ward or by any other form of useful productive activity, the better both for the patient and for his recovery from his illness. Illness to the young child may represent a traumatic and punitive separation from the home. To the older adult, illness may be perceived as a worrying disablement. To the young adolescent, however, illness is usually accepted as a temporary setback which must be conquered as soon as possible, and in this sense the adolescent patient is most likely to co-operate with the nursing and medical staff to ensure a speedy recovery.

The Adolescent as a Nurse

Many readers of this book will be student nurses who are themselves in the late adolescent age group. Other readers who are already trained nurses working in a supervisory capacity will be responsible for the handling and training of student nurses. It is, then, perhaps pertinent that we should finally consider some of the problems of adolescence as they affect the young person who begins training as a student nurse. As Mrs N. MacKenzie has pointed out in her excellent article on 'The Personality of the Student Nurse' (1945), those concerned with nursing training must remember that many of the difficulties which arise will be due to the fact that the nurse in training is, at one and the same time, a student who must be taught, a nurse who must carry out nursing duties and, finally, an adolescent. Our previous comments on the adolescent personality are, of course, equally applicable to the young man or woman who enters nursing during this period of development, and there is no need for us to repeat our earlier observations. The specialized vocational role of the modern nurse, however, raises certain specific issues which are not equally relevant to adolescence in general and it will be our purpose here to review briefly some of these issues.

At a period of life when the young person is most conscious of himself and often wishing to have more privacy a vocation which involves a system of communal training is bound to create some problem of adjustment. This applies to all adolescents who start work for the first time. In a way it can be compared to the child's earlier task of adjusting himself to the group life of schooling. This point is, however, particularly relevant in the case of the student nurse who must also learn to adjust herself to a set of fairly rigid traditions and rules. The nurse might also be resident in the hospital and, therefore, have to adjust herself not only to communal training but to communal living. Living and working as one of a group containing people of different and often opposing outlooks and opinions is, of course, a valuable socializing experience but, nevertheless, it does create difficulties. Some adolescents will equally find their social role in the nursing group in the same way as some children have no difficulty in fitting themselves in to their school group. Others, who are more sensitive and less sure of themselves, will adjust themselves more gradually and perhaps with more difficulty. In some cases the young man or woman may resent this intrusion in their privacy and find it difficult to reconcile their own needs and habits with the often divergent views of their new colleagues. Some time in life we must all learn to make a working balance between the things we would like to do and the inconveniences our behaviour would cause to others, so this aspect of communal living provides a very useful training for life itself. We have already seen that most adolescents have a strong desire to assert their individuality and to be accepted as self-reliant persons in their own right. Although often uncertain and unsure of themselves they are particularly sensitive to being treated as children or to being placed in any situation which curbs their natural assertiveness. The young nurse of to-day no longer has to adapt herself to a rigid and inflexible set of rules and regulations which governed the life of nurses in the past. Some senior nurses no doubt regret the passing of many of the more strict forms of regimentation which at one time made the nurse's training days comparable with the experiences of the new recruit in the army. At the same time there is little doubt that even to-day the young nurse must adapt herself to a discipline which is more demanding and often more inhibiting than that which faces the young person taking up a vocation in, let us say, the commercial or industrial world. Again, there is little doubt that this discipline which, amongst other things, teaches the young nurse a code of manners and general conduct is, in many respects, highly beneficial in inducing a more adult responsible outlook. Most young nurses who take a pride in their work and who have a respect for their nursing superiors will take this discipline in their stride. In fact, like the young child, they will often welcome a sensible and rational code of discipline which offers them much needed security and guidance. There is little doubt, however, that at times the right to discipline the student nurse is abused and that the short-sighted and high-handed attitudes of some senior nurses provoke only a rebellious attitude on the part of the nurse. Some time ago I was attending a nursing conference. On returning to the afternoon session, in which I was presenting a paper, I found that I was a few minutes late. I was soon reminded of this by being met at the door by a very forbidding looking senior nurse who, thinking that I was a nurse, questioned me in detail as to where I had been and treated me to a long lecture. There is no doubt, of course, that I had committed a breach of courtesy by my lateness, but the objectionable feature of this incident was the attitude of the senior nurse which implied that I was a young child who had been naughty and would have to be chastised. If training is to be successful the nurse must have achieved at its completion an ability to use her own initiative and to think and act like a mature adult. Naturally enough, if the nurse is treated repeatedly as if she were a child this will have the reverse effect. We can, in fact, again compare our views here to our views of discipline in childhood. Sensibly applied discipline will allow the nurse to retain her self-respect and by appealing to her reason will allow the nurse to incorporate these rules within her own personality so that the final result will be one of voluntary self-discipline.

We would, of course, be led far astray if we took all the student nurse's reactions in her training at their face value as being merely her reactions to the present situation. The emotional and other problems which face most adolescents in one form or another will naturally affect their work and the student nurse might be expected to transfer and displace many of her own problems into her vocational life. To take one obvious example, if a young girl is having difficulties at home in her relationship with her parents her emotional reactions to this situation may affect her work as a student nurse. All of us tend at times to make our jobs the scapegoat for our personal troubles and there is little doubt that many of the complaints one might hear from nurses in reality represent their reaction to personal problems which have nothing to do with nursing. Ideally, any person whose job it is to control and direct the young nurse in her work must consider each nurse as a person who has a life outside the hospital wards which may well affect her behaviour inside the ward. This does not mean, of course, that the ward sister and other staff should intrude in the nurses' private lives but only that they may be misled and frustrated in their training capacity if they completely ignore such external influences on the nurses' behaviour. Earlier we drew attention to the range and depth of feeling which is characteristic of the young person and makes him more emotionally vulnerable to certain situations. In their day-to-day work student nurses will be constantly faced with birth, illness, suffering, and even death. They must, if they are to become efficient nurses, learn to view such experiences objectively while at the same time remaining sensitive and sympathetic to the feelings of patients and relatives. This delicately balanced attitude is a difficult one to attain and can only come through experience. For some time the young adolescent nurse may find herself easily upset by what is going on around her. The older, more experienced, nurse who may have forgotten her own earlier reactions may find it difficult to understand or appreciate this situation and may become a little impatient with her junior colleague. The young nurse in her turn must often mistakenly regard the more objective and matter-of-fact attitude of the trained nurse as indicating callousness and a lack of regard for human life. Although the young nurse can only reach a more balanced view through experience, those responsible for training can again greatly facilitate her task by their sympathetic understanding of the factors involved.

One of the chief responsibilities of those in charge of student nurses is that of relaying to them the knowledge and specialized techniques of nursing. In a later chapter we will be considering the learning process in more detail and here we are concerned only with the impact of adolescent experience on the student nurse's training. Most young people during adolescence are enthusiastic and eager to learn as much of the world around them as possible. They are unsure of themselves, conscious of their own ignorance, and anxious to translate their inexperience into the experience and knowledge which will give them the confidence they so urgently need. The older nurse who has already been concerned with the training of student nurses may feel that this is an over-optimistic and idealistic impression of the attitude of the student nurse to her work. We must remember, of course, that the young person's eagerness to learn may be hidden by shyness, brashness, or even a show of cynicism. The young person often learns by bitter experience that her rather clumsy and unsophisticated enthusiasm provokes only amusement or derision from the adults around her and she may defend herself from being hurt in this way by adopting an outward 'couldn't care less' attitude. None of us like to be made to look foolish in the eyes of others, but the adolescent with her extreme selfconsciousness is more than ordinarily sensitive to the embarrassment of this type of situation. Those responsible for training the student nurse, then, must take this into account and avoid a public show of the young nurse's mistakes. This may seem largely a matter of common sense but too often one does find that senior nurses tend to overlook the harm done by using the inexperience of one young nurse to further the experience of others in the ward or classroom. Later, we will be considering some of the technical and academic aspects of the ward sister's role as a teacher in relation to the student nurse. In doing this we must not forget that one of the most important functions of the ward sister is that she will automatically function as a model with whom the young nurse might identify herself. We have already seen that the impressionable adolescent soon looks for new heroes outside the family group and certainly many a young nurse's total attitude towards nursing is largely modelled upon her first experiences with figures in authority such as the ward sister. In other words, the ward sister's personality is perhaps as important a determinant in the training of the student nurse as is her technical skill and abilities. There is nothing more shattering to the idealistic student nurse than to be faced by a cynical older nurse who, by her general attitude and actions, creates a sense of disillusionment which destroys the student's wholehearted enthusiasm and makes her vocation 'just another job.' During the rather turbulent passage of adolescence the young person searches for something which will give her life a meaning and purpose and allow her to express herself in relation to others. The young person who becomes a student nurse is fortunate in that she has entered a vocational field which does offer an opportunity of endowing her life with productive and satisfying work. It is again the responsibility of those in charge of training to see that the young nurse's early training experiences are rich enough to allow her a sense of achievement, a gradual feeling of self-confidence, and pride in her work, and above all, the knowledge that she is participating in what can be the most satisfying of all human activities, the alleviation of human suffering.

In her very interesting and informative book, *Psychology, the Nurse and the Patient* (1954), Doris Odlum has this to say of the nurse's vocation: 'The career of the nurse or doctor certainly does involve considerable personal sacrifices, but the work itself is so interesting, so essentially worth while, and brings such tremendous rewards if one does it well, that it is worth making sacrifices for. One must feel that one is dedicated to it. You cannot do it in the spirit that you would do shorthand or typewriting, or some such mechanical job. Anyone who wants to work in that way should not take up nursing, but those who are prepared to make the sacrifices and who have the sense of dedication will, I am sure, find that they are living a life of great fulfilment.' Perhaps it is worth adding one more comment to Miss Odlum's description. The phrase 'dedicated nurse' too often suggests to people a picture of a man or woman whose whole outlook and, indeed, whose whole life is narrowly centred upon their career in nursing to the exclusion of all normal human pursuits. Nothing can be farther from the truth. Any nurse who is correctly trained and has been able to extract the full benefits of her working role as a nurse will have achieved not only success in her job but success in developing her personality. The fulfilment which comes from a sense of responsibility to oneself and others brings with it an inner maturity which affects the nurse's life outside as well as inside the hospital. The good nurse is a complete person who also makes a good citizen, a good friend, a good wife, and a good mother. The experiences of nursing bring with them an acceptance and understanding of oneself and others which is the hallmark of the mature adult and the key to a well-rounded and satisfying life.

Concluding Remarks

In our review of adolescence it may be thought that we have over-emphasized the difficulties inherent in this phase of development. It is certainly true that many adolescents, judged on the basis of their behaviour alone, seem to experience few of the problems which we have mentioned. This, of course, does not deny that the young person may be experiencing all the inner uncertainties, fears, and doubts which are a natural consequence of the changes which take place during this period. Again, we might say that many adolescents do not have the insight or experience to formulate and express the feelings which are aroused and which, to a large extent, dictate their behaviour.

At present one reads and hears of many well informed and knowledgeable adults who express grave concern regarding the state of youth in the world today. The older man or woman is bewildered by the fads and fancies and general activities which currently occupy the majority of young people. Probably one of the first signs that one is growing old and rigid in one's thinking is when one finds it impossible to identify oneself with young people and to understand their outlook. In most of us, no matter our true age, there is a little of the child left and a great deal of the adolescent. It is when we turn our backs on our own early enthusiasms, our hopes, our day-dreams, and our ideals, that we cease to understand the new generation and begin to grow old within ourselves. The habits of youth in each generation tend to be criticized and derided by the youth of the past generation who, now older but not always wiser, have preferred to forget their own past experiences. John Raven (1952), dealing with this question in his book *Human Nature*, quotes the following passage: 'The world is passing through troubled times. The young people have no reverence for their parents; they are impatient of all restraint; they talk as if they alone knew everything, and what passes for wisdom with us is foolishness for them.' This might have been written today but it is reassuring to find that in actual fact it was said by Peter the Hermit during the eleventh century. Finally, let us remember that the values or lack of values which we find in the youth of today are in one sense a reflection of the faith and system of values of the adult world. The young person developing towards maturity must adjust himself to many new situations. Perhaps the most difficult bridge he has to cross is that between the social role of the child and that of the adult. To a large extent adolescence represents an apprenticeship for manhood or womanhood and, like all apprenticeships, it demands training, experience, and constant guidance. The adolescent should qualify at the end of this apprenticeship as an adult in the full sense of the word who is able to accept himself and develop his individual gifts to their best advantage. The attainment of such a qualification is, however, by no means an automatic consequence of reaching the age where one is accepted as an adult citizen. As we shall see, many individuals remain adolescents for the rest of their life and are never able to attain the inner wisdom and self-acceptance of full psychological maturity.

QUESTIONS

1. Discuss some of the difficulties which may face the boy or girl passing through the adolescent phase. Do you consider any of these problems to be unavoidable? If so, what form of advice might benefit adolescents and their parents in making this period of life less troublesome?

2. What are the principal psychological disorders which may occur during adolescence? Comment on the degree to which these disorders are a reaction against the social role of the adolescent in our own society.

3. What are the main differences you might expect in the adolescent's reaction to illness and hospitalization as compared with the reaction of the younger child?

4. Describe some of the ways in which the adolescent nurse might benefit, as a person, from nursing training.

3. Adulthood

Although a legal age for the onset of adulthood is easily decided it is less simple to denote its psychological onset. Adulthood carries with it a certain level of maturity that is not a necessary consequence of reaching any particular age. To some extent the criteria of mature adulthood have already been implied in our discussion of adolescence. Maturity involves a realistic adjustment, both to the environment and to one's self. By achieving insight into one's own limitations and potentialities we learn to accept the former and develop the latter. We turn aside from the unattainable day-dream and employ our energies in a more realistic striving for the attainable. We learn to accept the responsibility for our actions, make our own decisions and learn by our mistakes. Gradually we learn to accept responsibility for others, this reaching its full development as the young adult himself becomes a parent.

Problems of Adulthood

As it is obviously impossible for us to consider the many psychological problems which confront adults, we shall confine ourselves to a brief survey of some of the broader areas of stress.

1. Work

We have already stressed the human need to find a purpose and significance in life and certainly work offers one situation in which the adult might hope to find such a sense of purpose and achievement. Most of us are firmly entrenched in a specific vocation long before we are of adult age, for our choice of career is decided during adolescence. The ideal here, of course, would be that each person finds the type of work to which their individual talents, abilities, and interests are most suited. Unfortunately, this is far from the case and many people spend their working life doing something for which they are comparatively unsuited. In such a position the individual is often unable to achieve any real satisfaction and work provides a means of living rather than providing a meaningful living. Nowadays schools, commerce, industry, and professions combine with such bodies as the Ministry of Education to ensure that as few square pegs as possible land in round holes. This type of vocational guidance and selection serves an extremely useful function but is too often ignored or given only a cursory glance. Even with the best guidance we are still faced with the unpleasant conclusion that, in a modern industrial society, many people must occupy jobs which are uninteresting and certainly lacking in the sense of purpose and achievement enjoyed by the creative craftsman of the past. Whatever the tribulations of nursing, the young man or woman who enters this career can be sure of the opportunity of working in a field which offers unlimited scope for achievement, purpose, and personal satisfaction. Many people who are less fortunate in their vocation achieve the same sense of satisfaction in their activity outside work, whether it be in the garden, in the home, in their social life, or in their hobbies. Only too often, however, we find that the person who is bored at work is also bored when not working. With the gradual shortening of the working week one of our society's future problems is to aid people in finding more satisfaction in their increasing leisure time. A man or woman who has a passive and mentally inactive role at work tends to be equally passive and inactive in leisure. The future paradise of a twenty-hour working week loses its attraction if we visualize half the population spending the remaining hours gazing apathetically and bleary-eyed at their television screens. The only answer to this vast social problem lies in education orientated at developing wider, more creative and social interests, a 'do-it-yourself' policy which is easier to conceive than to put into practice.

Even to those who are reasonably suited for their jobs, work still creates many problems. Most of these problems arise from the necessarily competitive nature of work. Most of us like to have a sense of advancement in our work, seeing ourselves make steady progress up the ladder of promotion and vocational success. In any competition there must be losers and thus many adults feel frustrated and embittered by their lack of progress. Others, by dint of great effort and determination, rise to higher positions above the level of their true abilities, but only at great personal sacrifice. I remember one young business man who craved promotion but reacted with vague gastric symptoms and severe backaches to every occasion when promotion seemed a possibility. He sensed that a higher position would put too great a strain on his intellectual resources and he feared also the increased responsibility which promotion would bring. Success is hollow if it includes a gastric ulcer or an inability to enjoy life. We return again to the question of insight, for the mature adult is able to gear his aspirations to his personal capacities. In work, as in all of life, he finds his own level and obtains satisfaction in the knowledge that he is doing his job well. Given a reasonable chance the able person will overcome obstacles at work and reach the top, while others less suited and unable to accept their particular limitations will feel cheated and envious.

It has been said, in reference to nursing, that the 'good' nurse seldom becomes the 'successful' nurse, the implication being that the nurse who enjoys working with patients finds little interest or attraction in administration. It is easy to detect a 'sour grapes' flavour in this type of remark and it would be perhaps more correct if we altered the sense of the comment a little to say that the successful nurse is simply the nurse who gets the most out of (and puts the most into) her work. In 1955 a team of investigators studied the day-to-day work of mental nurses working in the Manchester area. Their conclusions are specifically levelled at mental nursing but their closing lines are of equal application to all types of nursing. 'It is important to remember, too, that, in the eyes of the patient, the status of the nurse is not determined by the nature of the work—the grade or rank held—but by the personality and attitude of the individual' (Manchester University, 1955).

2. Courtship and Marriage

The adult faces not only the problem of selecting the right career but also the right marriage partner. Although we do have marriage guidance councils which might be compared to the vocational guidance councils it fortunately remains true that science has not yet advanced to the stage where we could have a scientific assessment and selection of marriage partners. Perhaps the day will come when we shall be paired off according to our brain patterns or metabolic rate but as yet we are thankfully allowed to make our own mistakes. During late adolescence young men and women are attracted to each other in a predominantly physical way although this may be garlanded in romantic ideals. As age advances the adult is still attracted by the physical desirability of the opposite sex, but now the qualities of companionship become increasingly important and the boy friend or girl friend is valued according to the pleasure and satisfaction their company brings. Ideally, marriage should involve both a physical attraction and a respect and genuine bond of fellowship between the partners. This is the difference between loving and being in love. The word 'respect' above is important, for too often a marriage fails because of the inability of either partner to respect the other's individual integrity. Some people marry with an idealized picture of their partner which bears little relation to the person he or she actually is. Faced later with the reality of the situation the husband or wife either feels cheated and disillusioned or thereafter endeavours to manipulate their partner into becoming the person of their illusions. Two people cannot remain married for long without both of them changing in their outlook and habits as they adapt themselves to each other's ways, but there is a limit to such adaptation. No person can have their personality changed and remoulded to suit the demands of another and the result must be mutual disappointment and antagonism. Other immature adults seek to re-establish in marriage the security and lack of responsibility of childhood. Unconsciouly, they seek not a husband or wife but a father or mother and they marry someone who resembles in appearance or in some aspect of their personality the parent whom they still need. Again, this type of union is unlikely to result in a happy marriage for no man or woman can live up to this dual role and achieve happiness with a husband or wife who is unable to assume the responsibilities of married life. Successful marriage is built upon the capacity to share experiences, both pleasurable and unpleasurable, while still respecting each other's right to an independence of personality and spirit. Life shared in this way can be doubly satisfying but the capacity to share and to understand must be equally present.

It is not surprising that most surveys of marital problems agree that the success of a marriage is likely to be impaired if one of the two partners is neurotically disturbed. A number of such surveys have observed that where one partner shows evidence of personality disorder there is an increased likelihood of the other partner also suffering from neurotic tendencies. This observation might reflect a tendency for neurotically inclined people to seek out and marry partners of a similarly nervous disposition. A possible alternative explanation is that sharing one's life with an emotionally disturbed person is likely to cause an initially stable partner to become nervously disturbed. The available evidence (Kreitman *et al.*, 1970) seems to weigh on the side of the latter explanation, in that husbands or wives married to a neurotic partner are usually found to be normally stable early in the marriage, but to become increasingly neurotic with successive years of marriage. One study (Nelson *et al.*, 1970) comes up with the interesting finding that, in a marriage where either husband or wife are neurotic, the partners tend to spend more time in each other's company than in marriages with a low incidence of personality disorders. Such findings might prompt the cynical conclusion that mental health in marriage is enhanced by the partners avoiding too much of each other's company!

Although the physical side of married life is only a part of the whole, it does symbolize the basic feelings upon which the marriage rests. It represents an experience which should ideally be equally shared and involve mutual respect and understanding. If this aspect of married life is not mutually satisfying it is almost certain that the whole marriage will fall short of what it could be. The young people of today are infinitely more knowledgeable about sex and their own bodies than any past generation and certainly one of the greatest enemies of marital adjustment is fear and ignorance. Given this basic knowledge, however, the success of the physical relationship will merely reflect the underlying mental attitudes which decide the success of the marriage as a whole.

The maintenance of a perfectly balanced sexual partnership throughout a long-lasting marriage is perhaps unrealistic. The many other demands of marital life are bound at times to interfere with sexual compatibility. Successful marriages are able to survive the inevitable differences in sexual satisfaction by the good natured tolerance which comes from mutual respect. A rather amusing example of one man's reaction to the strains of marriage upon sexual harmony is contained in the following letter quote in Dominion's (1968) book on *Marriage and Marital Breakdown*:

To my ever-loving wife,

During the past year I have attempted to seduce you 365 times. I succeeded thirty-six times. This averages once every ten days; the following is a list of excuses on the unsuccessful occasions:

We will wake the children	7
It's too hot	15

It's too cold	3
Too tired	19
It's too late	16
It's too early	9
Pretending to sleep	33
Windows open, neighbours will hear	3
Your back ached	16
Toothache	2
Headache	26
Giggling fit	2
I've had too much	4
Not in the mood	21
The baby is crying	18
Watched late show	7
Watched early show	5
Mudpack on	12
Grease on face	6
Reading Sunday Paper	10
You are too drunk	9
We have company in the next room	7
Your parents were staying with us	5
My parents were staying with us	5
Is that all you ever think about?	105

Do you think you could improve our record this coming year?

Your ever-loving husband

A very experienced psychiatrist once said to me: 'Many marriages fail because people expect too much of marriage.' This statement may at first sound cynical but it contains an essential and important truth. No two people can share all the everyday demands of life without at times crossing swords in violent opposition. The wife or husband who boasts that 'we have never had a cross word' is usually either forgetful or sitting on a time-bomb. Marriage, like all human activities, demands constant adjustments and it is unreasonable to assume that such adjustments can be made without some measure of disagreement. Where there is mutual respect and understanding, however, both partners can afford to be themselves and know that differing opinions will not threaten their bond.

Before leaving the topic of marriage, it may be interesting to observe that the true attitudes of today's teenagers regarding marriage may be somewhat different from that reflected in popular stereotypes concerning young people. In a carefully conducted survey of almost 2,000 English teenagers, Schonfield (1968) found that only 4·5 per cent of boys and 1 per cent of the girls interviewed rejected the concept of marriage as it concerned their own future. The same survey demonstrated that the average teenager was a great deal less sexually sophisticated than is often assumed and that many of their attitudes on family, social and moral issues were surprisingly like those of their parents. Perhaps the generation gap is not as great a yawning chasm as we have been led to believe.

In today's world marriage is obviously no longer the predominantly permanent liaison which it was in the past when divorce was more difficult to obtain and socially disapproved. One might feel that the more flexible nature of marriage today is a great improvement on the over-rigid bonds of the past. It might be argued that the lessons learned from one disastrous marriage will increase the possibility of a succeeding marriage being successful. However, the facts would appear to contradict such an assumption. Dominian (1968) quotes the following data from one American study. The separation and divorce rate of first marriages was found to be 16·6 per cent; where one partner had made a second marriage the rate rose to 36·8 per cent; when both partners had been married twice before, it rose to 79·8 per cent. Apparently marriage does not improve with experience.

3. Parenthood

While the achievement of a successful marriage represents one of the chief signs of maturity, it is probably true to say that an adequate adjustment to parenthood is of even more importance. If this psychological hurdle is overcome with little disturbance we can be fairly certain that the adult has arrived at full maturity. Modern methods of birth control have changed the act of having a family from what was once an automatic function to one which can be deliberately planned or avoided. There are now very few people who do not possess the knowledge of family planning and most psychologists would agree that the advantages of this social change by far outweigh the disadvantages. The process of child-birth is a natural biological function which, given reasonable physical health, should involve little difficulty. Unfortunately, child-bearing is still too often shrouded in mystery, ignorance, and fear in the minds of many people. Sometimes this is due to faulty education and misunderstanding regarding the normal functioning of the body. More often it is due to less rational but more powerful feelings of which the person herself is not fully aware. Some women reject pregnancy because of unhealthy attitudes created by their own parents, some because they associate pregnancy with pain rather than joy, and others because of an inability to accept their adult responsibilities. This last factor may also prevent the husband from accepting parenthood. If he married only to secure, rather than to share, affection he may see a family as a burden or even a rival for his wife's attention. During pregnancy itself an enormous amount of anxiety and mental agony is created again by lack of knowledge or by the many childish fantasies which surround childbirth. The mother to be may worry that her child will be born deformed, that she may injure the child during pregnancy, that the unborn child may cause her suffering or even death, and a host of other irrational fears. The father to be may feel rejected, particularly if his wife cannot accept him sexually in an erroneous belief that this might injure the child. The father may even so identify himself with his wife that he takes upon himself the symptoms of pregnancy. Every doctor is familiar with the male patient who develops backache, gastric pains, constipation, and so forth during his wife's pregnancy. Finally the actual process of the birth itself may be made more difficult by the frightened mother whose tenseness impedes nature and causes the very pain which she fears. As we have already commented, some of these reactions to childbearing are the result of deep-seated fears which are resistant to rational explanation. A great many of these reactions are, however, produced solely by misunderstanding and ignorance, and such fears may be evaporated by advice and explanation. The nurse working in the pre-natal clinic or the maternity ward is well qualified to pass on her own knowledge and experience to the parents and so help to remove the worry and tension from an event which should be gratifying and joyful. The nurse should not wait for the parents to express their difficulties in direct questions for many of them are ashamed or afraid to expose their ignorance and misconceptions. Instead the parents should be offered spontaneous explanation and be encouraged by the sympathetic understanding of the nurse to air their fears.

Often the real problem of adjustment comes after the actual birth when both parents have to readjust their way of life to fit in with the demands of the new member of the family. Parenthood brings with it new responsibilities, new restrictions, and new differences of opinion which again test any marriage. The husband may feel that he is being overlooked by the busy mother who may, in her turn, feel that nature has made an unfair division of labour between the sexes. Many difficulties can be solved by the parents working together and as far as possible sharing the new responsibilities. Letting father bath baby may take twice as long and cause temporary chaos but it does help to unite the family (and perhaps teaches the bewildered infant to swim). There are many other problems raised by parenthood as the child develops but we have dealt with most of these in our earlier discussion on the child in the family and therefore need not concern ourselves with them here. It may be worth while to remind ourselves that the problems of parenthood are far outweighed by the joy and happiness of this most important of human functions.

4. Loss of Loved Ones

Most young parents themselves still possess parents and it is the eventual loss of one's own parents which involves the next stressful situation which faces all adults. The immature adult who has never been psychologically 'weaned' from his parents is still dependent upon them to a great extent and the realization of their advancing years, their approaching and subsequent death, represents an acute problem in their lives. Even the more mature adult suffers a profound psychological disturbance at the loss of his parents. Again, people react in a variety of ways to such loss. Some are able to express their natural grief and so learn to live with the reality of the situation, while others are deeply affected but are unable to accept completely the full implications or obtain relief by expressing their feelings. The reaction will, of course, depend greatly on the age of the parent, the age of the adult, and the general circumstances. The effects will probably tend to be less severe if the adult is married and able to share his or her feelings with an understanding partner. Perhaps the greatest measure of comfort is, however, to be found in the act of the adult achieving parenthood for the advent of a new generation symbolized by the child creates a feeling of immortality and, to some extent, compensates for the loss. One of the most important but most difficult tasks in rearing a family is in helping the children to become as independent of the parents as is possible. The more dependency the parent creates the more pain and suffering will be caused by the inevitable parental loss. Perhaps one of the nurse's difficult and unpleasant tasks is in dealing with bereaved relatives. There is little really concrete that she can offer but the helpful comfort of her understanding of the feelings which have been aroused.

5. Growing Older

The later part of adult life, the period of middle-age, also creates new problems which demand new adjustments from adults of both sexes. By this time families have grown up to become independent and have left the parental home. It is often as difficult for the parents to learn to become independent of their children as the children of the parents, and many middle-aged parents find their life growing emptier as they see their children marrying and building their own lives. The appearance of grandchildren helps to make amends and fill the emotional gap which has been created. By middle-age most adult have a fund of experience which can be applied in new interests outside the home and many people find a new lease of life in taking a more active part in community and civic life. The increased leisure time which comes with middle-age allows a general widening of interests and many people find that they are now able to do many things which were not possible before. In this way the later period of adulthood can be extremely stimulating and enjoyable. Too often, however, the parents have invested themselves too deeply and too completely in the rearing of their children and find it difficult to adjust themselves to the change in their situation. This might apply particularly to middle-aged women who, after a long period of being tied to the home and family, find middle-age creating a vacuum which they lack the flexibility and initiative to fill. When taking out insurance to cover themselves in their later years, most adults would be advised to insure themselves also against future boredom and loneliness by maintaining active interests outside the home.

Middle-age also involves a variety of physiological changes which demand psychological adjustment. A general decline in physical capacities, although gradual, usually becomes apparent in middle-age and forces the adult to make some limitations in physical activity. There is little doubt that the middle-age 'change of life' contains more implications for the female adult as compared to the male. The menopause which occurs in women between the mid-forties and fifties denotes a physiological change of which the most direct effect is inactivity of the reproductive processes. The resulting disturbance of the endocrine balance produces the familiar symptoms of flushing, dizziness, sleeplessness, and general excitability. It is difficult, however, to distinguish between the direct effects of the physiological changes and the indirect effects of the individual's psychological reactions to them. It is generally agreed that many of the disturbances which are frequently associated with the menopausal period are indirect and unnecessary consequences of the feelings and attitudes aroused at this time of life. Here again the knowledge and experience of the nurse can act as a valuable antidote to the undesirable products of the menopause. Replacing ignorance with fact can give the middle-aged woman a more confident understanding of the changes which are affecting her body. However, the real answer to many of the problems which affect both sexes at this time of life lies in a broad adult education which will aid the older adult to make a confident adjustment by demonstrating the new interests and enjoyment in life to be found in middle-age.

Standards of Normality

In preceding pages we have referred to the terms *normal* and *abnormal* but have not yet defined their meaning. Like many words in both everyday and technical usage, *normality* is given many shades of meaning. Perhaps the most common lay use is exemplified in the words of an American comedian who declared: 'My wife is abnormally immature, if I'm sitting peacefully in my bath she'll think nothing of walking right in and sinking all my little boats!' In this usage it is assumed that we are normal and that the behaviour of others may be judged abnormal to the extent to which it deviates from our own standards. Normality as a psychological concept has at least four different meanings, some of which have uncomfortably much in common with that expressed above.

The Dichotomous Concept

The history of psychiatry has involved much argument between those who measure mental health on a continuum and those who regard normality and abnormality as constituting a clear-cut dichotomy. In medieval times the latter view was well accepted. People were either healthy and normal or abnormal and possessed by a devil. Although this view has been greatly modified with increased understanding of mental illness it was not until the advent of psychoanalytic theory that the dichotomy between normality and abnormality was finally bridged. By viewing neurotic symptoms as a product of unconscious conflict Freud demonstrated that the difference between normality and neurosis is one of degree and not of kind. Although few contemporary psychiatrists disagree with this argument as applied to the neuroses the dichotomous standard of normality is still often applied in the case of the more serious psychotic mental disorders. The conception of specific disease entities which has dominated European psychiatry since the time of Kraepelin denies that the psychotic process is merely an extension of normality. A person has or has not schizophrenia, just as he has or has not cancer. It is now appreciated that this all-or-one concept cannot always be correctly applied to physical illness and it may well be that the dichotomous approach may have to be abandoned in psychiatry. However, at the present time we do have two separate standards of normality operating in the field of mental health, depending upon the nature of the disorder. This double standard easily leads to double-talk in psychiatric diagnosis when we fail to distinguish which standard is being applied.

The Statistical Concept

In discussing the distribution and measurement of intelligence a purely statistical approach to normality is utilized. Normal intelligence is here defined as being around an I.Q. of 100 and abnormal degrees of intelligence, low and high, lie on either side of the distribution curve. The *normal* may be the *average* in many aspects of human behaviour and this is an assumption used by the clinical psychologist in assessing mental health. This way of assessing normality is quite different from the dichotomous approach, for it implies a continuum between normality and abnormality, which differ only in degree. The whole idea of constructing standard psychological tests of behaviour is based upon a statistical approach to normality and in practice this often works well. A statement that a one-year-old infant's physical development is abnormal because it deviates in certain ways from the average level of development of other similarly aged infants is informative and useful. The parallel statement that a person's behaviour is abnormal because it deviates from the behaviour of others of a similar age and background is also useful but a great deal less simple to demonstrate. While it is relatively easy to assess the normal (average) level of physical development at different ages it is extremely difficult to assess what is the normal distribution of specific forms of behaviour. Another difficulty is that the norm of behaviour may vary in different social groups. If a statistical survey of the incidence of wife-beating is made it will be found to occur sufficiently infrequently to call it abnormal behaviour. However, if the survey is confined to a particular social group it may be found to be statistically normal for this sample. Are we then to say that for members of this social group it is abnormal not to beat one's wife? This dilemma is perhaps more evident when we consider the third concept of normality.

The Adjustive Concept

A common denominator in all mental disorders is the inability of the individual to adjust harmoniously to others and to the society to which he belongs. Thus a common criterion of normality in psychiatry is the degree to which an individual is able to adjust to his environment. Inability to accept the prevailing social standards, either because of aggressive defiance, fear, withdrawal, or personal deficiency, becomes the criterion of abnormality. This method of defining normality equates it with conventionality. The well-adjusted person is the conventional individual who conforms to the prevailing standards of conduct. This approach has much in common with the statistical method, both equating unusual and unconventional behaviour with abnormality. This concept of normality has provoked the caustic comment that 'the capacity to share the delusions of the crowd is a sign of individual health'. If normality is measured in terms of adjustment to society, it is clear that mental health must be assessed with reference to a particular society. An individual, who is well adjusted and therefore normal in one society, may be maladjusted and abnormal in another society. As different cultural groups with differing standards exist within any one society, the decision as to whether an individual's behaviour is to be judged normal or abnormal requires detailed reference to his social background.

This problem is often intensified by the fact that those who have to makes such judgements (psychiatrists, social workers and magistrates) are frequently from a different social background from the individual whose normality is to be assessed. In some parts of the Scottish Highlands 'second sight' is not so much a sign of abnormal mental functioning as a matter of keeping up with the McDonalds!

The Ideal Concept

Some systems of measurement are based upon a flawless or ideal standard of normality. If the dentist used a statistical concept of normality he would remove healthy teeth in an effort to make his patient more 'normal' for his age. The dentist and the physician have in their mind an ideal set of teeth and a perfectly functioning human body which, although seldom seen, act as a standard of normality. Unlike the other views, the ideal concept implies an absolute, rather than a relative criterion of normality. Although this approach avoids many of the pitfalls inherent in the other concepts it is seldom used in psychology. The reason for this is simply lack of adequate knowledge of the ideal qualities of human behaviour and mental health. Perhaps one day understanding of human nature will be sufficiently advanced to allow us to aim at an ideal level in human behaviour.

Psychological Disorders in Adulthood

Many of the common psychological disorders of adult life may be viewed as reactions to the problems we have been discussing. Mental ill-health is the failure of the individual to adjust himself to current stress. Its cause then is to be found in the constitutional and psychological make-up of the individual which predisposes him to breakdown or in the degree of environmental stress to which he is subjected. In most cases both these factors operate in producing the disorder.

The most common explanation of the neurotic symptoms offered by adult patients who attend psychiatric out-patient departments is that of overwork or of stress associated with their work. Often this is merely a rationalization, it being easier and more comforting to find the reason for one's 'nerves' in something external like work than to admit that the true causes lie inside one's own personality. However, a person's work may be directly related to the neurotic ailments which affect so many adults in the community. If we are unable to achieve a sense of satisfaction and purpose from our work we are to some extent thwarted in expressing ourselves, with resulting feelings of inner dissatisfaction and frustration. The same situation may result if, lacking sufficient self-insight, we allow too great a gulf between our ambitions and possible attainments. If our hopes and aspirations are beyond our capabilities we will be haunted with a sense of inner discontent simply because we have set ourselves tasks which we cannot possibly fulfil.

We have already referred to the new adjustments which every adult has to make when faced with the responsibilities of marriage. Once again the individual reactions to marital experiences will depend both on the degree of actual stress imposed and the individual's capacity to cope with such stress. One of the most common sources of anxiety, particularly during the early part of marriage, is the sexual adjustment.

Ignorance or mistaken ideas regarding sex on the part of one or both of the marriage partners may make what should be a natural expression of mutual love a traumatic and frustrating experience. Early failure to achieve a satisfactory sexual relationship may cause undue anxiety which in turn inhibits the individual's natural feelings resulting in a vicious circle of repeated anxiety and frustration. Such experience, in the case of the sensitive individual, may cause general symptoms of impotence in the male and frigidity in the female. Fear of pregnancy may also underlie sexual anxiety although modern methods of birth control greatly minimize conscious worry of this order. In many psychological disturbances of a sexual origin 'treatment' takes the form of direct education to give the individual a more rational and less erroneous conception of sexual matters. Where the sexual disturbance is but a symptom of a more general and deep-seated anxiety the problem may prove more resistant to direct instruction and require a more intensive psychotherapeutic approach.

Another common time of psychological disturbance is during pregnancy and after childbirth. We have already referred to the emotional disturbances which sometimes affect both the male or female adult during the childbearing period. The period following the actual birth of the child is also associated with psychological illness which is sometimes of a more serious nature. The combination of psychological and physiological changes which occur at this time make most women susceptible to emotional upset and it is relatively common for the new mother to feel rather disturbed and depressed for a short time after the baby is born. In the great majority of cases this mood soon gives way to one of pleasure as the mother quickly adapts herself to the new experience. Certainly she may remain a little more excitable and emotional for some time, but she gradually settles down to a normal tempo. In a few cases, however, the disturbance is deeper and more long-lasting. Symptoms such as anxiety or depression may persist to such an extent as to make the mother unable to cope with the increased demands in the home and cause her to feel extremely unhappy and ill at ease. When the nervous symptoms reach the point of causing an actual breakdown in the patient's capacity to lead a normal life some form of treatment is desirable. Pregnancy and childbirth involve a number of physical and mental changes and treatment here will depend upon the cause of the disturbance. Some form of psychotherapy is usually advisable for the cause of the nervous breakdown may lie in unconscious emotional conflicts, induced by the experience of having a child. In a very small proportion of cases the disturbance may be so profound as to constitute a *puerperal psychosis*. A few of these states are toxic in origin and related to puerperal fever but the vast majority fall into the two major categories of schizophrenic and affective (depressive) psychoses. We have already described schizophrenia as it arises more commonly in adolescence or early adult life and the symptoms of puerperal schizophrenia are similar although the nature of the illness may be at first masked by a general picture of delirium. Affective psychosis usually takes the form of a severe depression with symptoms of deep despair, feelings of acute hopelessness, hallucinatory experiences, and a general retardation of the patient's thoughts and movements. Patients suffering from puerperal psychoses are invariably treated with the physical therapies applied to psychiatric illnesses in general, *i.e.*, insulin coma therapy in the case of schizophrenia and electro-convulsive therapy in the case of depression. The actual cause of a psychotic illness during the puerperium is far from clear. The variety of endocrine and metabolic changes which take place probably make their contribution, but it is unlikely that these changes alone could produce a psychosis of the same type as occurs more commonly outside the puerperium. We are forced to adopt the more general explanation that certain individuals are constitutionally predisposed towards psychotic breakdown in the face of stress. Childbirth involves some degree of physiological and psychological stress and this may 'trigger off' the latent psychosis.

The nurse can play an important role in the psychological disturbances associated with pregnancy and childbirth. By offering understanding and rational explanation she can help to replace the doubts and fears, which so often distort both the sexual relationship and childbirth, with confidence and insight. By her appreciation of the emotional state of the mother following the birth of the child she can help to make the situation less traumatic and disturbing and greatly reduce the likelihood of long-lasting anxiety. Finally, with her knowledge of the more serious peurperal illnesses, she can observe and report any suggestive symptoms which become noticeable while the patient is still in hospital and thus draw early attention to the patient's condition.

Another major area of psychological disturbance in adult life is the period of middle-age. The new adjustments which have to be made at this time may again result in psychological disturbance. Each individual will react in his or her personal way and the symptoms again may vary from subjective feelings of anxiety, depression, or general tension to somatic disorders which have an emotional root. If a psychiatrist had to select one psychological symptom which is most characteristic of breakdown in middle-age he would undoubtedly choose the symptom of depression. As age increases our emotional reactions to stress appear to be coloured by feelings of sadness and depression.

Earlier we named schizophrenia and the *affective psychoses* as being the two major categories of psychotic illness. Although schizophrenia is more likely to show itself in adolescence, affective disorders usually begin to be clearly apparent during early or late adulthood. This difference in time of onset between the two forms of psychotic illness is, however, by no means the rule and the decision to consider them here separately, under the headings of adolescence and adulthood, is to some extent an arbitrary one. As the term implies, the affective psychoses are disorders which effect primarily the mood state of the individual. Depression is the most common form of disturbed mood and we have already referred to reactive depression in speaking of neurotic disorder. In reactive depression there is usually a fairly clear-cut precipitating event which has occurred recently and which can be linked with the onset of the depressive symptoms. In the case of many people who suffer from a depressive illness, there is however little or no evidence of any events occurring in the environment which might have triggered off the subsequent depression. Indeed some depressive attacks appear to have no causal connection with events outside of the patient, giving the appearance of having arisen from within the patient himself. Psychiatrists refer to this type of depressive illness as *endogenous depression* and it is thought that such depressive attacks are caused by internal biochemical changes which are themselves constitutionally determined. This division of depressive illnesses into the reactive and endogenous types is, however, fraught with confusion and is in itself probably responsible for a great many of the ambiguities which occur in psychiatric diagnosis. It will be evident from our earlier discussions that every form of human behaviour, whether it be healthy or pathological, must involve both the individual's constitution and his environmental experience. We might well ask why the same type of environmental experience causes some people to respond with a reactive depression, others with neurotic symptoms, while some are able to adjust normally to the experience. A probable answer is that people are constitutionally predisposed to react to environmental stress in different ways and in different degrees. It seems equally unrealistic to imagine that, in endogenous depression, the patient's experiences and the environmental stresses to which he has been exposed have no influence in initiating the depression. We know by experience that a patient who has been successfully treated for an endogenous depression will have a much better future prognosis if he or she is returning to an environment which is not too stress-provoking. It might then be more realistic if we thought of depressive illnesses as being arranged along a continuum, characterized at one end by purely endogenous reactions based on constitutional factors alone, and at the other end by purely psychogenic reactions to environmental stress. Most people who suffer from a depressive illness could probably be placed somewhere near the middle of this continuum, thus indicating that their illness was determined by a complex mixture of constitutional and psychogenic factors. It is nevertheless true that some individuals who present with a neurotic reactive depression have undergone such a degree of stress in their personal environment that their resultant symptoms seem to be almost entirely a psychogenic reaction. It is also true that there are some patients whose depressive illness appears to be almost entirely endogenous and unconnected with events in their environment. The best known of these predominantly endogenous affective disorders is that of *manic depressive psychosis* which includes within it the two apparently opposite poles of disordered feeling, mania, and depression. At one time mania and depression were considered to be two quite separate types of illness until Kraepelin was able to demonstrate that they formed a single disease process, characterized by the extreme affective states of elation and depression. In the course of this illness some patients alternate between the two extremes of mania and profound depression, with intervening periods of normality. Others suffer chiefly from either mania or depression, showing only very short periods of the opposite affective state. Within the affective state itself the degree of disturbance can also vary a great deal. Thus the manic phase of an affective disorder may vary from mild hypomania to severe and acute mania. In hypomania the patient is over-active in his behaviour, variable in attention, and lacking in patience. In his mood he appears over-cheerful, animated, subject to fleeting enthusiasm, but is likely to respond with irritation or aggression to any frustration or delay. The mood state of such patients may appear highly enviable but their constant cheerfulness, the superficiality of their feelings and the pressure of their talk and activity soon becomes wearing to anyone who is in their company for any length of time. As the manic mood heightens and passes into the more acute manic state, the patient's behaviour becomes more uncontrolled. The pressure of speech and thinking speeds up until the patient may become quite incoherent and unable to attend to anything for more than a few seconds at a time. The patient becomes more and more over-active and his sleep is likely to be grossly disturbed. In his mood he becomes increasingly elated and has no insight into his mental state, declaring himself to be feeling healthier than he has ever felt before. In the upper levels of mania the patient may become quite exalted and grandiose, believing himself to be of great importance. In their speech such patients often show the typical 'flight of ideas' in which the direction of thought is continually interrupted by their following up multiple associations to each word. At this point the patient's behaviour is usually quite bizarre and he may, for example, write meaningless messages to people of importance. At one time the fully exalted state of mania could be extremely dangerous for the patient, whose over-activity was likely to lead him to the point of physical exhaustion. Today, however acute mania may be terminated more easily by the application of the correct drugs or by the use of E.C.T.

The depressed phase of a manic-depressive illness may also vary from a simple depression to a depressive stupor. In its milder form, depression is characterized by the general slowing down of physical and mental processes so that the patient is retarded in all his responses. Indeed the patient's first complaints may be that he is not able to get through the same amount of work, or if a housewife, that she is unable to cope with her usual domestic routine. In his mood the depressed patient feels dejected, pessimistic about the future, and he may become preoccupied in a morbid way with his own health. He finds his interests waning and his attention can no longer be held by activities which he once enjoyed. He feels the world is a miserable place and cannot visualize either future improvements or remember a time when he felt cheerful and content. His appetite becomes disturbed and he begins to lose weight. Sleep is nearly always impaired, the most frequent complaint being of wakening in the early hours of the morning and being unable to get back to sleep again. As the depression develops the patient becomes more retarded, feels more dejected and may become preoccupied with feelings of guilt and unworthiness. The patient may feel that his present state is a just punishment for past misdeeds, the significance of which he now greatly enlarges in his mind. The unpleasantness of his state may be heightened by the development of strange feelings of depersonalization and derealization and at this stage the patient may become quite deluded and out of touch with reality. In the extreme state, the depressed patient can lose all apparent touch with the outside world, becoming quite stuporose and unresponsive. It is obvious that in all depressive illnesses the risk of suicide is always present, and it is therefore important that depression should be diagnosed and treated as early as possible.

The majority of patients suffering from a manic-depressive disorder tend to suffer from periodic attacks of either mania or depression although, as already stated, some patients show an illness which pursues a more cyclical course, embracing both elation and depression. The specific causes of this disorder are not yet fully understood but there seems little doubt that a biochemical disturbance plays an important role in the genesis of depressive illness. Studies of heredity also indicate that there is a large genetic component particularly in the case of patients whose illness pursues a regular cyclical course. In recent years the lives of many individuals with a manic-depressive history have been almost miraculously changed by the discovery that lithium salts injected in regulated doses may interrupt the manic-depressive cycle and prevent the occurrence of future attacks.

Another common form of mental illness of the middle-aged period is *involutional melancholia*, so named because of its association with the endocrine and metabolic changes of the climacteric (the so called 'change of life'). The symptoms of this illness are traditionally held to be somewhat different from that found in depression at other stages of life, but some studies (Tait *et al.*, 1957) suggest that such differences have been greatly exaggerated. Most of the symptoms are certainly indistinguishable from that of other forms of depression. The illness usually begins with complaints of fatigue, lack of energy, and general retardation. Sleep is disturbed, with early morning wakening being typical and the patient loses his appetite. The mood change develops from mild depression into a state of utter dejection and misery, and again the patient becomes preoccupied with feelings of guilt. Depression occurring in the involutional period is usually thought to contain a higher incidence of hypochondriacal symptoms of a bizarre nature. Thus the patient may become convinced that his insides are rotting away, his bowels are blocked, or that his stomach is being eaten by worms. Hallucinations are also thought to be somewhat more common in involutional melancholia than in other forms of depression and agitation and anxiety is another familiar feature.

Any description of the symptoms of a depressive illness

paints a rather gloomy picture and, of course, the patient who is in a profound depression certainly presents a pitiful and wretched picture. Fortunately, however, this illness is one of the growing number of psychiatric disorders for which there is a specific and effective method of treatment. E.C.T. (electro-convulsive therapy) can bring about a surprisingly rapid improvement in the condition of depressed patients and the introduction of this treatment has allowed many patients to be discharged from hospital after a few weeks or months completely recovered. Now added to the range of available treatments for depression is a number of new pharmacological methods of treatment (the tricyclic preparations) the advantage of which is that the patient may be treated with such drugs without coming into hospital.

Once again we may comment on the similarity between this illness, in its milder stage, and states within normal experience. We have all known people who are habitually mildly hypomanic in nature and indeed in some occupations such a disposition might be a decided asset. There are others who suffer from spells of depression which are close to the milder forms of the depressive phase. Finally, there are many people, well within the orbit of normality, who are variable in mood and tend to fluctuate between elation and mild depression. This link between normal behaviour and mental illness, which we have noted before, probably explains in part the fear, and sometimes intolerance, of the mentally ill which is still present in society, in spite of our educational advances. It is only too easy at times to identify oneself with the patient's illness and some defend themselves against this realization by regarding the sufferer from mental illness as a creature from an alien world.

Psychological disorders, of a moderate or severe form, represent a gigantic and often underestimated social problem. More man-hours are lost to industry every year by adults suffering from nervous disabilities than by physical illnesses, strikes, or any other cause. It has been estimated that approximately one in four of adults who consult their general practitioner do so with disorders which are not solely physical in origin. Some of the disorders we have mentioned have undoubtedly a physiological basis but emotional factors also figure in all, though to a differing degree. The emotional problems which underlie many of these disturbances can be studied and treated psychologically but their aetiology is often a social and interpersonal one. When adults become adult enough to come to terms with themselves and each other, living socially and not merely in society, then perhaps there will be less need for psychiatric attention. The other evening I was watching a television programme on psychosomatic medicine, the closing words of which serve as an apt conclusion for our own discussion here. 'In this world today there are less people who are unhappy because they are ill than there are people who are ill because they are unhappy.'

Before leaving the topic of depression we might consider in a little more detail the problem of suicide, which is always a paramount danger in the handling of the depressed patient. Not all people who unsuccessfully or successfully attempt to take their own life are clinically depressed. However, depression probably lies at the root of most suicides. Curiously enough, the risk of suicide often is higher when the patient appears to be responding favourably to treatment and shows clinical improvement. One of the symptoms which commonly accompany the deepest levels of depression is *retardation*—a progressive sapping of one's energy level and an inability to initiate any activity. In the retarded state, the depressed patient almost literally lacks the initiative to seek an end to his misery in suicide. The medication which will eventually alleviate his depressive mood sometimes first alleviates the level of retardation, before normalizing the mood state. It is at this paradoxical point of some improvement that suicidal behaviour may be more likely.

There are many dangerous myths connected with suicide. Thus, it is often said that people who talk about taking their lives or who make several abortive attempts will never really kill themselves. Nothing could be further from the truth. The vast majority of successful suicides occur after a history of repeated declarations of intent or unsuccessful bids, which are construed by others as being merely hysterical bids for attention. Indeed, individuals who suddenly and unexpectedly kill themselves without first emitting clear danger signals are very uncommon.

Suicide tends to have a higher incidence in certain segments of the population. People who are single, divorced, separated, living alone, or in any way socially isolated are more likely to commit suicide than those who are more fully integrated within society. Women make many more unsuccessful suicidal attempts than men but men outnumber women in successful attempts. This sex difference is probably related to the mode of suicide chosen, in that the male is more likely to utilize methods which are more likely to be deadly and irrevocable (e.g. firearms), while the female more commonly choses methods which allow more chance of intervention (e.g. drug overdose).

Over the last decade or so there has been a measurable increase in suicides in two discrete age groups—the old and the young. The longer life span resulting from advancements in medical science means that more people live into old age but, as we will argue in the next chapter, society has yet to make adequate provisions to ensure that these bonus years will be happy and fulfilling. Among the young, the most alarming increase has been in those who continue in higher, post-secondary education. University students show a much higher incidence of suicide than others in their age group. In one U.S.A. study (Seiden, 1966) suicide was the second most common cause of death in students, next only to accidents. Interestingly enough, the typical suicidal student is not one who is struggling in terms of academic performance, but rather one who shows a consistently high calibre performance. Typically, he is a chronic overachiever who is highly self-critical and never reassured by a repeated history of academic success.

The great pity in most cases of suicide is that this terrible waste of a human life is usually avoidable. As we have already stated, the danger signals are usually clearly evident. In many cases the underlying depression motivating the suicide would have responded to treatment if diagnosed in time. Anyone who gives any indication of suicidal thoughts must be taken as a potential threat to his own life.

The Adult as a Patient

The days are now gone (if they ever existed) when a patient coming into hospital was treated as a diseased liver, appendicitis, heart, etc., and not as a person. However, in the skill, time, and energy which goes into modern hospital treatment it is still only too easy to underestimate the importance of the patient as an individual. The patient's state of mind will also play some part in the response to treatment and, in some cases, it may take the leading role. Last year I saw a patient, suffering from a severe depressive illness, dying in hospital of an attack of influenza. The physician who fought to save her life remarked that the patient had no resistance and that she seemed to have 'no will to live'. This is by no means an uncommon happening. Many patients with mental illnesses die of physical ailments which a mentally fit and resilient person would throw off with ease. The human organism has an inborn capacity for self-preservation which allows it to react to disease in such a way as to repair the damage done as far as possible. Our blood clots over the wound, our broken bones knit together, our organs work more efficiently to compensate for a diseased organ. The physician may apply the means of cure but he depends on the body's normal working to ensure that his treatment will do its job. The way a patient feels in hospital, then, is important, not merely in an ethical but in a medical sense, for the state of mind may impede or promote recovery from illness. In this section we will consider some of the reactions of the adult patient to his illness and to being a patient in hospital.

The adult patient's reaction to illness will obviously depend mainly upon the nature of the illness but it will also be influenced by what the illness means to the patient. Medicine in the eyes of the public is a subject which is shrouded in mystery and a great deal of this mystery is an inevitable result of the complex nature of the subject itself. A contributing factor to public ignorance of illness, however, comes not from the subject itself but its practitioners. Many medical people feel that the less the public know about medical matters the better (as illustrated by the current outcry of the British Medical Association against television presentations of medical subjects). Naturally it would never do for the public to become too conversant with medical knowledge and we must agree that the publicity of such information is like fodder to the hypochondriacal adult who 'collects' symptoms. However, the worst anxiety and fear is usually that caused by ignorance and it is just this fear of the unknown which so often exaggerates the patient's reaction to his illness and its treatment. The normally intelligent adult is likely to benefit from some explanation of his illness and its implications. The patient is unlikely to remain in ignorance regarding his illness for long and the source from which he finally receives his information may be a much less satisfactory one. All nurses will be familiar with the informal symptom discussion groups which spring up between patients in every hospital ward. The more ignorance regarding the illness and treatment the more room there is for the ward patient to obtain a dangerous status in the eyes of his fellow patients by setting himself up as a misinformation bureau. The uncertain and anxious patient is also only too liable to seize upon odd remarks by the nursing and medical staff and to misinterpret them completely in line with his own fears. In a later section (Chapter 9) we shall deal in more detail with some other problems of communication in hospital which affect, not only the patients, but all staff members.

Whatever form his illness takes each adult will tend to react in some way to being hospitalized. Coming into hospital disrupts the patient's normal routine of living in a variety of ways but perhaps the most important of these changes is that the patient surrenders his adult independency to become greatly dependent upon others. This enforced dependency, combined with the fears aroused by illness, often results in the patient *regressing* in behaviour in so far as his reactions become less adult and more child-like. This regression may show itself in different ways. Some patients will become completely passive and over-dependent in their behaviour, doing practically nothing for themselves and demanding constant attention. Others will react with peevish, irritable, and irrational behaviour, like spoiled children, while yet others will become over-anxious, frightened, and seek continual reassurance. Each patient, in fact, will tend to react to the situation in terms of his or her individual way of reacting to past emergencies encountered in their earlier life. It is again important to remember that patients' behaviour, which may annoy the ward staff and increase the work, may represent not their normal personality but an emotional reaction to being in hospital. The more the patient's fears are allayed by reassurance and explanation the less will be the disruption in his normal behaviour.

We earlier referred to the fears which may be aroused in the child patient by unfamiliar surrounding, uniforms, and apparatus. Adult patients are no less susceptible to similar fears and, for example, what to the nurse is a simple routine examination may to the patient represent a terrifying ordeal. It is being more and more recognized that a few minutes' explanation of what the examination or treatment involves, before the actual procedure is carried out, is time well spent. If a certain amount of pain is expected to accompany any procedure it is usually better to inform the patient first. Nothing is more calculated to shock the patient and destroy confidence in the staff than the nurse who declares that 'this won't hurt a bit' before carrying out some procedure involving a fair degree of discomfort and pain. One cannot, of course, lay down general rules here, for each patient is a separate individual and the nurse must gauge her way of handling the patient on her knowledge of the personality of the patient. Some patients will have special phobias, such as a fear of injections, which will require individual attention. Where the patient's illness demands surgical intervention special problems may occur. Many adults who have little fear in respect of medical treatment react with considerable anxiety to surgical treatment. Our body and its organs are an important aspect of our 'self' and the suggestion of surgical treatment is liable to raise fears of deformity and internal disturbance. A number of studies of patients facing the stress of surgery provide vivid illustrations of the important role the patient's psychological state plays in his physical recovery from stress. In one U.S.A. study, patients awaiting major surgery were randomly allocated to what might be termed a 'fully informed' and a 'relatively informed' group. Patients in both groups were given a few basic facts about their approaching operation—such as when it would take place, the length of time involved, etc. In addition to such basic information, the 'fully informed' group were given a great deal of detail about the operation itself, instructions as to the post-operative aches and pains they might expect and other specific information of events likely to occur in the recovery period. The follow-up demonstrated that the informed group were not only significantly less anxious during the post-operative period, but also required less day and night sedation, made a better and quicker recovery and were able to be discharged from hospital earlier than the uninformed group. In essence, this represents another example of a common observation in stress studies. The greater the amount of specific information one possesses regarding any approaching stressful situation, the more one is able to mobilize one's individual defenses and personal coping strategies to reduce the eventual impact of the stress. It is perhaps plain from what we have been saying here that the efficient nurse can never be a completely dispassionate ministering angel. She must be able to effect the difficult compromise between a cool and objective attitude in her technical procedures and a warm personal and understanding attitude in her handling of the patient as a person. She must accept the fact that, although many of the patient's fears may appear foolish and irrational, they nevertheless cause suffering and discomfort which hinder the patient's progress. Many of the patient's fears will, of course, be perfectly rational and only indirectly related to hospitalization. Thus adults will tend to worry over personal problems such as the effect of their illness on their jobs, the welfare of the family who have been temporarily deprived of a parent, and so on. Naturally the nurse can hardly be expected to function as a welfare worker and almoner but again her awareness of the patient's state of mind and her sympathetic understanding of the patient's difficulties is in itself therapeutic.

Most adult patients gradually learn to adjust themselves to the new and often bewildering life in hospital. Although accepting the hospital routine, some aspects of it must seem baffling to the patient who cannot possibly realize the complex organization which necessitates many of the apparently unnecessary procedures. Recent years have seen a general loosening of some of the more traditional and less meaningful hospital procedures but there are still a few practices which are difficult to justify. An ex-patient complained to me ruefully that her most traumatic experience while in hospital was waking up at an unearthly hour in the morning to find herself already half washed by an efficient nurse.

The final point we might mention here is the problem which arises from the enforced immobility which often accompanies illness and hospitalization. The patient who is confined to bed and restricted in his general activity may turn his attention inwards on himself and become over-introspective. Such self-absorption may lead to a morbid and hypochondriacal over-attention to symptoms. The adult patient should be encouraged to remain as active and outgoing in his interests as is possible in order to combat the undesirable effects of such withdrawal.

The Adult as a Nurse

By the end of her training course the once inexperienced student nurse will have become the experienced and efficient qualified nurse. She will not only be no longer regarded as a student nurse in her working capacity but will now be regarded as having reached an adult status as a person. Her success as a nurse will depend not merely on the degree to which she has been able to digest the specialized and technical knowledge of her profession but also upon the degree of personal maturity she has attained. We have already referred to the following qualities as denoting adult maturity: insight, responsibility and self-reliance, integrity, a sense of purpose and emotional control. The ideal nurse possesses sufficient self-insight to enable her to form mature relationships with patients and colleagues which will not be unduly influenced by her personal difficulties. Having learned to accept and be at ease with herself she will have no difficulty in accepting and being at ease with others. She will be a reliable person with the self-confidence and initiative necessary not only to carry out the orders of her superiors efficiently but to arrive at her own decisions when circumstances demand. At the same time she will continue to learn both from the greater experience of others and from her own mistakes. Her personality will be sufficiently integrated to allow her to be herself at all times. In the course of her duties the nurse must interact not only with patients but with hospital colleagues in the nursing, medical, and administrative staffs serving in junior and senior capacities. Professional etiquette naturally demands that each member of the staff be given the respect due to them according to their rank and experience. The ward sister or staff nurse must necessarily adopt a somewhat different approach in her relations with senior medical and nursing staff than she adopts in her dealings with her junior colleagues. However, the nurse who, for example, demonstrates an excessively servile and submissive attitude to seniors and an excessively aggressive and dominating attitude to juniors will win little respect or confidence from anyone, patients or staff. The successful and adult nurse will also possess a sense of purpose and achievement in relation to her vocation and to life in general. She will find that whatever of herself she puts into her work is more than repaid by the satisfaction which she receives from doing a worth-while job well. Finally, she will have sufficient control over her feelings to enable her to approach every situation with an attitude of mind which is unbiased by emotional extremes but which is at the same time warm and sympathetic. The adult nurse who completes her training armed not only with the technical knowledge and information, which she learned in the classroom and in the wards, but with the strength of character developed by her experience, is likely to ascend the ladder of promotion. In Chapter 10 we will discuss more fully the functions of leadership and the personal qualities which distinguish the good ward sister or the efficient administrator.

Perhaps the reader may reflect a little caustically that the ideal nurse, as here described, exists only in the fancies of psychologists who have never themselves coped with ward nursing duties. Although lacking this corrective experience, the author has worked with many nurses who easily meet all the criteria of maturity which we have considered, although they themselves would be the last to admit this. Young men and women who 'grow up' in nursing have an excellent opportunity of eventually becoming more adult and mature than their fellows in other vocations. The ethics and values which are traditional in the nursing profession, the variety of experience, the day-to-day personal contacts, and, above all, the sense of working for the welfare of others, all combine to make the nursing role not only one of the most interesting but one of the most personally rewarding of occupations. The ideal adult is one who has ideals and the profession of nursing not only fosters and develops ideals but gives them a means of expression.

Concluding Remarks

Our main theme in this section has been that the development of the adult personality is not an automatic and inevitable process. The attainment of adult maturity is a consequence of the individual's experiences in adapting himself to his environment and the degree of maturity achieved will vary from one person to another. Some people will take longer than others to 'grow up' and become mature adults, while others will remain 'childish' and immature in their outlook and behaviour throughout their life. Maturity represents an attitude of mind rather than a stage of physiological development. Essentially it denotes a final discardment of the remnants of the egocentric attitude which dominates our childhood and the assumption of a more realistic and rational attitude to life. It is a process of coming to terms with ourselves, accepting our personal limitations, and at the same time developing our potentialities. The mature adult does not only make an end of self-deception but learns to accept and love others for what they are in themselves. This capacity for tolerance, respect, and acceptance of others brings with it a final independence. By realizing that the things which are important to us may be unimportant to others and the experiences which bring pleasure to others need not be the ones which bring us pleasure, we become self-reliant and independent. There is no longer any pressing need to conform and to be afraid of being 'different'. A middle-aged patient told me the other day that he had 'lived a compromise all my life between the person I wanted to be and the person others expected me to be'. Naturally we all have to make some the development of our own personality and causing us to lead an artificial existence then we are being dishonest, not only with others, but with ourselves. Personality traits have a wide and varied distribution and no two individuals can ever be identical in their natures. In social relationships, for example, some people are good talkers and others good listeners; some are good mixers while others are more shy and reserved; such differences of personality are disadvantageous only when they become a matter of concern to the individual who cannot enjoy being himself through his desire to become like others.

The greatest test of adult maturity is psychological stress. Adult life contains many problems and difficulties, some of which we have considered. If we are able to face these situations realistically, without self-deception or distortion, then we learn by our experiences and become a little more stable and mature. Parents have a natural protective desire to remove as much stress as possible from the lives of their children. They sometimes forget that, in shielding the child from life's obstacles, they are also denying the child the opportunity to cope with future stress by rising above present difficulties.

Like the young child, the immature adult is essentially self-centred. He is too occupied in dealing with his fears and inadequacies to be able to relate himself to others. The mature adult, in comparison, is at peace with himself and finds further fulfilment in his fellowship with others. The ability to love others unconditionally is not only a paramount feature of Christian belief but also the key to maturity. We might fittingly close this section with a second quotation from the writings of John MacMurray. 'Clearly, therefore, our capacity to realize our nature and to be ourselves in full achievement depends upon the extent to which love is the dominant motive of our total activity' (MacMurray, 1950).

QUESTIONS

1. Discuss the various meanings attached to the concept of normality.

2. To what extent might the nurse's appreciation of some of the problems faced by the average adult (man or woman) assist her in caring for the adult patient in hospital?

3. What types of situations in adult life might possibly precipitate some form of psychological disorder? Say how an understanding of the factors involved in such disorders might help to prevent or alleviate them.

4. What are the most important qualities which the ideal nurse should possess? Can you think of any aspects of the nurse's duties which are likely to encourage the development of such qualities in the trainee nurse?

4. Old Age

This final stage of human development has been the focal point of a great deal of psychological study in recent years. As a result of medical progress and greatly improved social conditions more people are surviving into old age and their welfare is one of today's most pressing social problems. How much of this task still remains to be done is to be seen in the high proportion of elderly people who today live in mental hospitals. This fact raises the important question of whether the psychological changes associated with old age are an inevitable part of the biology of ageing or are avoidable consequences of social organization. As with growing up, it is difficult to link the onset of old age with any specific chronological age. The sequence of physical and mental changes in later life differ greatly from one individual to another. Indeed, perhaps the most striking feature of ageing is its individual variability.

Earlier categorization of adolescent changes into their physical, mental and social aspects provides a useful framework in which to examine the changes of later life. A reduction in physical energy is accompanied by increasing dimness in vision and hearing. Alterations in muscular control reduce mobility and the speed and dexterity with which movements may be made. These and other physical changes have a common psychological consequence for the elderly person in restricting his former pursuits and limiting his social relationships.

The mental changes in old age are many and complex, which is another way of saying that we have still much to learn about them. There is a reduction in the capacity to learn new principles, resulting in a progressive dependency on principles and ideas learned in the past. The older person tends to be more rigid in his thinking, less able to adapt himself readily to new ideas and experiences. There is a demonstrable reduction in the capacity to handle information. It takes longer to grasp information and less can be held at any one time. Retention of information in the short-term is also easily disturbed by any other activity going on at the same time. These changes result in a tendency for the older person to be slower in grasp, poor in concentration and unreliable in his memory for recent events. Recall of events in the more remote past is seldom impaired, this being another factor in making the elderly person more comfortable and assured when dealing with the past rather than with the present. Earlier it was suggested that one of the hallmarks of successful development in late childhood was the capacity to control impulses and emotions. In old age there is often a noticeable decline in this control so that the old person may appear childish and over-emotional in his responses.

The social changes in old age reflect in large measure the role which society offers to its older citizens. Normally retirement from work occurs at the age of sixty-five although today people may still have many years of life ahead. It is not until retirement that people realize how dependent they have been on their work, even though their job may have been uncongenial or dull. Retirement involves separation from familiar surroundings and friends, and, most important, a negation of the lifelong pride of being an independent being contributing to society. It demands an abrupt change in established habits at a time when new adjustments are difficult to make. Such considerations do not similarly apply to the housewife whose job has no retirement age, although her own domestic routine is likely to be shattered by the continual presence of the breadwinner. The social status of the elderly person has changed considerably outside the setting of work. Grandfather is no longer accepted as the head of the family. Indeed, slackening of family ties may result in there being no easily accessible family contact. In this age with its emphasis on youth's speed and flexibility the elderly are not respected or revered, merely tolerated. Where once the elders advised and guided others they are now themselves being looked after by others. By being denied a viable functioning role the older person is made to feel a social liability rather than an asset. It is impossible to estimate how many of the less fortunate changes associated with ageing are a direct and avoidable result of the social vacuum in which many elderly people are placed. In societies where the elderly are still given a clearly defined and useful social role, there tends to be a lower incidence in the mental and emotional disturbances of old age.

Problems of Old Age

In this section we will concern ourselves with some of the problems which arise at this final period of human development. These problems can be viewed as reactions to the three categories of change which we have already outlined. Again, let us emphasize that there is no such individual as the average old person and that these problems and the individual's reaction to them will vary greatly, depending on the personal circumstances.

1. Work

The growing number of old people in the community has resulted in a number of psychological investigations into the capacities of the aged. These have confirmed the observations that older people tend to be slower in mental grasp and less capable in tasks demanding new learning. A number of these studies have shown, however, that quite minor modifications in the nature of the work task can often allow the older person to handle the situation adequately. Overloading of the individual's mental capacity would be more likely to occur in work demanding rapid responses to complex stimuli on where the job was being timed or paced by some external criteria. Often the older worker may demonstrate qualities which compensate for a possible decrease in the quantity of work output. He may be more conscientious in his attitude to work, more careful and certainly more practised. In most fields of modern industrial society, however, the retiral age is laid down somewhere in the sixties. At this time the man who has spent his life working is expected suddenly to adjust himself to retirement. If he has been fortunate and wise enough to prepare for his eventual retirement by creating for himself a wide field of interests to which he can devote his time, his retirement may give him a new lease of life. However, to many workers retirement means being cut off from familiar surroundings and friends and being relegated to sitting around the home or playing dominoes at the local old men's club. The sudden change in their routine not unnaturally makes them feel insecure and lacking in a sense of useful activity. These considerations do not apply so much to the woman who is fortunate or unfortunate enough to have a job for which there is no retiral age. Pensions and other provisions made by the welfare state do much to make up for the financial loss which retirement entails, although such arrangements are by no means all that they might be. In spite of what we may believe when younger, however, man's reaction to retirement usually confirms that we do not work merely for a weekly wage but that through time our work, and all that goes with it, becomes an integral and even indispensable part of our life. Even if we agree that modern economic and industrial conditions make it imperative that the older worker be replaced by his younger counterpart it would still seem that society has an obligation to provide the older person with some sort of opportunity to continue to be productive. It would not seem to be difficult to find many useful occupations to which the old person's undoubted assistance and experience could be creditably applied. It is, in fact, unnecessary for us to speak in terms of society's obligation because the old person has often still a great deal he can contribute towards society.

2. Interests

It is widely recognized that a person's interests change both in quantity and in quality in old age. Not unnaturally, interest in physical activities tends to decrease with age. In their place older people tend to become more interested in doing odd jobs in the home, reading, and enjoying entertainment such as the television, where they can take a less active role. It has also been found that older people tend to return to amusements and interests which are more solitary in contrast to interests which involve contact with others. Although the change in interests in old age is obviously connected with the decline in physical ability it is undoubtedly influenced by social factors. The reversion to solitary interests, for example, may be forced upon the old person by enforced isolation rather than represent a deliberate turning away from social interests. Unfortunately, many of the interests and hobbies which the older person could take up in later life are denied them by physical changes, such as failing eyesight or any of the mental changes which we have described. Denied their normal work and hobbies old people sometimes lack the knowledge or adaptability to turn to other pursuits and they relapse into apathy and boredom.

3. Isolation and Loneliness

Many factors combine to isolate the old person from others. Physically, old people are less able to join in activities involving effort. The gradual decline in the quality of the sense organs resulting in deafness, failing eyesight, and so forth, causes a further sense of being cut off from other people. The deterioration in the quality of intellectual output often makes it difficult for the old person to adapt himself to new ways of thinking and the new trends of other generations. The falling off in attention and concentration combined with poor memory for recent events tend to make thinking appear rigid and repetitive. He appears to be living in the past rather than the present. This is true to some extent, but his present difficulties and his lack of contact with present trends may be throwing him back to the past for consolation. If the old person is bored in himself he may be doubly boring to younger people around him who become tired and impatient of his incessant and repetitive talk of past glories and apparent lack of understanding of present day issues. Another factor which increases isolation at this time is the social change, particularly the loosening of family ties. If the old person is living with relatives he may be tolerated but seldom respected. More often than not he may be isolated in a literal sense in that he is living alone. There is little doubt that the prime problem of old age is loneliness. Recently the British Broadcasting Corporation carried out an excellent survey of old age and again and again the old people interviewed pathetically spoke of their extreme loneliness. Homes for old people would seem to be a partial answer to this problem, but this often represents to the old person a surrender of the only thing they have left, their independence. Many special clubs now exist for old people and they do excellent work in bringing the lonely together and so helping to dissipate their loneliness and much more of this type of work is needed. What many old people really need, however, is a feeling of being wanted. It is unlikely that institutions such as hospitals and clubs can ever meet this want, which can only be fulfilled ultimately by society's recognition that the old person can still play a positive and useful part in life. In my own work I see old people as patients in mental hospitals who crave only love and affection. In hospital they are well looked after but it is obviously impossible to answer their real need. In their behaviour they may sometimes be a little eccentric and not always easy to handle. At times they will be difficult to live with but one cannot escape the conclusion that their difficulties are enlarged by the refusal of the family and society as a whole to give them the understanding, affection, and respect which they have earned.

4. Disinhibition

During the first part of our life we tend to have little control over our feelings. One of the signs that adult status has been achieved is that the individual has gained control over his feelings and is able to inhibit emotional extremes. As age advances this capacity to control feelings by our reason weakens and the old person tends to be less inhibited in behaviour. In this sense old people often appear to be childish in that their feelings are aroused easily and excessively. Minor frustrations which would have been accepted at an earlier stage of life arouse intense feelings and they may react with outbursts of anger, rage, or 'huffiness' to events which seem to us trivial. They may also be extremely moved by small acts of kindness, responding with an embarrassing excess of gratitude and affection. As in children these feelings which are aroused may be fleeting and someone may be an object of their extreme affection one minute only to be regarded with scorn and derision the next minute. Again, like children, old people are apt to be 'naughty' in their behaviour, their moral sense becoming elastic to fit the occasion. I remember an amusing experience some years ago when one old man in hospital lost his false teeth. He was convinced that they had been stolen by a fellow patient and his response was to steal the set of teeth belonging to another old man in the ward. The second patient reacted in kind and, in no time at all, the nursing staff had to deal with a ward full of old toothless men who could not eat. It was only with great difficulty that things were sorted out and a fantastic teeth-fitting session resulted in order being re-established. In extreme cases, where the disinhibiting effects of normal ageing are exaggerated by senile changes, the lack of effective control may result in the old person clashing with society. I once interviewed a charming old gentleman of 86 years who had an irresistible impulse to pinch the bottoms of young ladies while travelling in public transport. He was otherwise perfectly charming and well mannered and his proudest possession was a magnificent collection of pin-up photographs. The forgetfulness and decline in control of the old person may sometimes result in a deterioration in personal habits. Less attention may be paid to eating habits and to general hygiene. This falling off of self-respect and social graces tends to be more evident when the old person lives alone and once again it is often difficult to distinguish between personality changes due to ageing itself and changes which are a reaction to being deprived of social attention.

5. Mood Changes

The physiological changes in the brain and nervous system occurring in old age may account for some aspects of the old person's behaviour. However, a great deal of behaviour of the old person may be viewed, as we have just suggested, as a reaction to the difficulties encountered. Every person does not accept with good grace the restrictions upon their activities and self-sufficiency imposed by old age. It is perhaps not unnatural that some should react with irritability and complaints which may appear unwarranted. Others may become unhappy and depressed over their inability to adjust themselves to a new and restricted life. Yet others, particularly those who are severely incapacitated by defects such as deafness in their ability to participate in what is going on around them, may become excessively suspicious and resentful of others. A final emotional reaction to the limitations imposed by advancing years is that of withdrawal of interest from the outside world with a corresponding increase in self-preoccupation. The more the old person feels cut off from the main stream of life the more he will tend to retire into himself. This may take the form of endless ruminations on the past or the development of a hypochondriacal attitude with constant complaining about aches and pains. To the outside observer the old person may appear to be full of self-pity and to show a selfish disregard for others. Although this judgment may be partly valid we must remember that old people retire into themselves only when forced to do this by circumstances. Some of these circumstances may be an inherent part of the ageing process but many of them are avoidable results of the lack of interest of society.

6. The Role of Faith

One of the ways in which the human race is distinguished from all other animals is in its capacity to be aware of its own mortality. We are conscious of the fact that all life is limited and that some day we shall all die. Our realization of this affects our lives in a variety of indirect ways but the full implications may not be felt until our span of life is nearing its completion. People vary in their capacity to adjust themselves to and accept the inevitable fact that life must end. The 'running-down' of the physical and mental processes in later life probably allows the old person to view the end with less distaste and apprehension than might the younger adult. There is little doubt, however, that a secure faith is the most powerful armament against a fear of death. Old age is very much a period where religious feelings are revived and strengthened. The inner conviction that death represents not an end but a new beginning allows the individual to anticipate the close of life with calmness and serenity. Others who lack religious faith may obtain comfort from their sense of having lived a full purposeful life. If one can feel that one has become what was in one to become by having fully developed one's personal potentialities then one has obtained a means of adjusting oneself to the last adventure.

Psychological Disorders in Old Age

Mental illness in old age presents an important and ever-growing problem to psychiatry. It has been estimated that something in the nature of between a quarter and a third of all admissions to mental hospitals are of people over the age of 60. That this is a growing problem is emphasized by the steady increase in the number of elderly people in the community. The falling birth-rate and the increasing span of life combine to cause a constantly higher proportion of old people living in the community. On this basis alone we would expect a larger proportion of old people to suffer mental illness and to enter mental hospitals for treatment. It does seem unlikely, however, that the increase in population alone can explain the much higher incidence in mental disorders of the aged at the present time. As we have already indicated it would seem quite reasonable to assume that another causal factor here is the lack of adequate social provision to meet the needs of the elderly person. The one factor of loneliness alone is enough to explain a great deal of the psychological disorders which affect the aged. Working in a mental hospital one cannot help but feel that the loosening of family ties and the decrease in the sense of individual responsibility present in modern society often cause families to look to the State and its hospitals to care for elderly relatives whom they find difficult to handle. It is, of course, only too easy for the outsider to be sentimental and idealistic regarding the fate of the elderly person who has become somewhat eccentric in behaviour. One must remember that the presence of a senile relative in a house may be a very disturbing factor and that the present generation of adults and children also have a right to live their lives without being unduly harassed by nursing the often difficult and demanding elderly relative. There is no doubt at all that many of these patients require the careful supervision and nursing which only the hospital can give but there are also a great number whose illness is much less acute and on whom hospitalization has a detrimental effect.

At one time it was assumed that the vast majority of old people coming in to mental hospitals could be classified as suffering from *senile dementia* subdivided into the two categories of senile and arteriosclerotic psychoses. Although the symptoms in these cases can be compared to a greatly speeded up and exaggerated pattern of the results of normal ageing, the general picture is quite different. The pathological disturbance of attention, memory, and thinking may be quite gross and the patient may be living in a self-made world to the extent of having lost touch with reality. By attending to the patient's physical health and helping to organize his daily life so that it is fairly settled and devoid of stressful situations we can help in alleviating the symptoms to some extent. However, there is no direct method of treatment here and no possibility of cure.

Post-mortem electromicroscopic examination of the brains of senile patients indicates a high number of 'senile plaques' —clusters of atrophied brain cells. The high correlation between the number of such plaques after death with the degree of behavioural deficit prior to death leaves little doubt that the deterioration in functioning is a direct result of the physical decaying process in the brain and central nervous system. However, it is also clear that socio-psychological factors may play an important role in deciding how incapacitating the physical process is to the individual's everyday behaviour. Thus, some elderly people who show quite advanced senile brain atrophy show less behavioural deterioration than might be expected, if they continue to enjoy the acceptance and support of their family and immediate neighbourhood.

In recent years, however, it has been demonstrated that a large number of mentally ill old people are suffering, not from an organic deterioration of the brain, but from a *depressive illness*. Estimates vary but it has been suggested that around half of the elderly cases of mental disorder fall into this category. The distinction between a psychotic condition which is depressive in origin and one which is due to senile changes is an important one, for the outlook in the former case is much brighter. Unless the patient's physical condition is extremely poor, depression in old age can be treated by electro-convulsive therapy with very good results. Modern developments in anaesthesia greatly limit the dangers of applying this treatment to the very old person and a large proportion of elderly patients are now able to return to the community and take up their normal life. While it is undoubtedly true that the old person's experiences have some effect upon the ageing process and even upon the pattern produced by senility, the environmental effect is of much greater importance in the case of depressive illness. It would seem likely that the elderly person who has been able to make a good adjustment to advancing years and who is still in active contact with other members of the community runs less danger of depression. The same may be said of prognosis as the chances of a good recovery are greatly increased if the old person has something for which to get well. A useful and enjoyable occupation, the love and affection of relatives, lack of financial difficulties, and a general retention of interest in life are all factors which one might consider as indicating a good prognosis.

There are other disorders which sometimes lead to the old person entering a mental hospital. Many of these involve a mental illness which is only an indirect consequence of physical conditions such as heart disease, brain tumours, or other infectious conditions. However, the number of such cases is very small in comparison with the number of old people who enter hospital with symptoms of either a senile or affective disorder.

The Old Person as a Patient

The old person in hospital presents a number of special problems which we might briefly consider. The first consequence of hospitalization is that it disturbs the patient's normal day-to-day routine. While the normal adult may adapt himself fairly easily to this break from routine, and may even rather welcome it, the elderly patient usually finds adjustment difficult. Many old people manage to make an adequate adjustment to their declining abilities by re-ordering their life around a rigid pattern of routine. Finding it difficult to deal with new or unexpected events they try to create a life where they can get by adequately by relying on well-established habits and set patterns of reaction. Each hour of the day is fitted into a carefully planned programme which resists change and avoids the unexpected. Coming into hospital represents an abrupt disruption of their normal routine which has provided an anchor of security and the old person may react to this with anxiety and perplexity. One of the first necessities in the nursing of the elderly in hospital is to answer the patient's need for a secure and well ordered existence. Fortunately hospital life is founded on systematic routine and the patients may learn to depend upon this regular pattern of activities as they once did upon their normal home routine. It may take them some time, however, to make the new adjustment and at first they may be awkward and difficult patients. A very real danger here, however, is that the patient's routine may become static. An elderly bed patient presents certain nursing difficulties but these difficulties may be much less than is the case when the patient is up and about. Today the emphasis is on keeping the elderly patient as mobile and active as possible thus avoiding stiffening and atrophy of the limbs through disuse. We have already referred to the dangers of mental inactivity resulting in withdrawal of attention and interest in the environment. Mental deterioration certainly tends to proceed more rapidly if the patient is immobile and inactive. The modern hospital ward with its facilities of radio and television and its occupational therapy department prevents the patient sinking into static inactivity. Of prime importance, however, is the patient's need for personal attention. Old people, like children, often make demanding patients in that they crave the reassurance, sympathy, and companionship of others. The nurse could easily spend her whole day merely listening to the patients, for they dearly love to talk to an interested audience. Although this is obviously impossible some time can usually be found for chatting to the patients and most old people have a great deal to say that is of interest. It possibly goes without saying that the elderly patient usually benefits from as much visiting as is possible without exhausting the patient. (Often it is the visitors who are exhausted first!)

We likened the nursing of old people to that of children in so far as they both demand attention. There are many other aspects where these two categories of patients present similar problems. Like a child, the old person's feelings are easily aroused and in both cases their behaviour will not always be rational. Petty jealousies, outbursts of temper, stubbornness, and all the other reactions typical of the very young patient can be seen again in the behaviour of the very old. If handled with tact and understanding most of these reactions are easily overcome, whereas a forcible and domineering manner may only serve to increase the patient's resistance. The nurse must, in fact, be prepared to spend a little of her time 'humouring' the elderly patient who is inclined to be resistant and difficult. At the same time we must desist from drawing our comparison too far. Although often 'childish' the elderly patient is not a child but an adult with a lifetime of experience. Most old people are particularly averse to being treated with jocular condescension.

Hospitalization represents more than a disturbance of the old person's normal routine. It also involves their surrender of what is often their most important possession, their independence. Most old people take a fierce pride in remaining independent as much as is possible. Their upbringing and general outlook make them averse to accepting charity and they are often suspicious of any assistance which encroaches upon their privacy and involves them in being dependent upon others. When, through illness or infirmity, they are forced to come into hospital this represents a final and complete intrusion on their privacy and their self-reliance. In hospital they are placed in a position of involuntary dependency for even their simplest needs. The patient may react to this situation with truculence and aggression which appears to the nurse as denoting ingratitude for all that is being done for their comfort and welfare. Others must react by yielding up all their initiative to become passively over-dependent upon the hospital staff. It is again vital that the nurse should have insight into the real causes of such reactions and not judge the patient's unco-operative behaviour at its face value.

Although having no direct experience of nursing aged patients I have worked with many old people in the course of normal clinical duties and in research projects of ageing. I think that most nurses who have nursed old people will agree that, although often demanding and difficult, they have many endearing qualities. One would have to be very cold and distant to avoid the spontaneous bonds of affection which spring up in one's relationship with these patients. One would also have to be supremely egotistical not to recognize that we have much to learn from them. They enrich us by their experience and they so often humble us by their pride, self-reliance, and independent spirit.

Concluding Remarks

The main conclusion at which one arrives through considering this final stage of man's development is that many of the personality changes we associate with old age are in reality reactions to the attitudes of society. It seems a short-sighted policy to ensure that man can enjoy a longer life while denying him the means of enjoyment. It is not altogether an over-statement to say that we as adults, by our attitude, tend to make people old before their time. There is a great need for social reorganization which will permit the elderly man and woman to continue to play a useful role in the community. As already pointed out, such provision need not be based on charity or social conscience alone as the old person possesses many talents which can benefit and enrich society as a whole. We have perhaps understated the fact that many old people achieve a stable adjustment and find that, like any other period of life, old age contains many benefits. Such people have usually led a full rounded life and have had the foresight to take with them into their old age a wide variety of interests. A very old lady was once asked by the author for her recipe for what was clearly to her a long and happy life. She replied simply: 'An open and inquiring mind, meeting new people, and a pint of stout a day.' Her last recommendation is perhaps a matter of personal preference but her first two suggestions are certainly worthy of universal application. An inquiring and lively mind which finds life full of interest depends for its development primarily upon education. Perhaps our educational system has tended to concentrate too much upon transmitting information and too little upon the more difficult task of fostering a healthy attitude towards the world around us. When people can find as much interest and reward in their leisure activities as in the narrower spheres of their work then perhaps there will be less need for society to ask itself: 'What shall we do about the old age problem?'

QUESTIONS

1. What are the main problems which face the aged in modern society? Distinguish between the avoidable and the unavoidable consequences of old age, commenting on any steps which might be taken to increase the sense of wellbeing of the old age group.

2. The two main psychological disorders of old age are senile dementia and depression. What are the most important differences between these two disorders with regard to prevention, treatment, and prognosis?

3. Comment on some of the nursing problems which might arise in caring for the old person in hospital. To what extent are such problems comparable to those which arise in nursing young children?

Part Two
Human Motivation

We have completed a very brief survey of the psychological implications of human development. From a consideration of how people behave we now turn to the related subject of what makes them behave in the way they do. In the following chapters we will be concerned with the forces which motivate human behaviour and cause us to act in specific ways. Knowledge of these underlying motives not only aids us in understanding the conduct of others but increases our appreciation of the true meaning and significance of our own actions. In the present chapter we will first consider the question of instinctive motivation before going on to comment briefly on the influence of our attitudes and emotions on our conduct.

5. Instincts, Attitudes, and Emotions

Instincts and Behaviour

Like many terms in psychology, the word 'instinctive' appears in different forms in our every-day speech. Thus we hear people say that they did something 'instinctively' or, alternatively, that they knew something 'instinctively.' By this they usually mean to convey that their action or thought was without any conscious deliberation and also that, to some extent, it was the correct thing to do or the correct conclusion at which to arrive. This meaning has much in common with the psychological meaning of the term 'instinct.' Instinctive behaviour describes, fundamentally, patterns of behaviour which are biologically useful, inherited, do not need to be learned, and require no conscious deliberation.

Numerous examples of instinctive behaviour can be seen in the behaviour of lower animals and insects. Species of sea crabs, for example, after birth automatically begin to march in the direction of the sea. Their journey is a hazardous one and the majority may die or be killed *en route*. They have had no means of learning this pattern of activity which compels them to act in this rigid manner. In the case of many creatures it is only necessary to learn their limited instinctive repertoire to be able to predict exactly how they will behave in any situation. In animals instinctive behaviour is characterized by its rigidity and lack of modification, the lack of learning, the uniformity of behaviour among the species, and the apparent absence of any awareness on the part of the animal as to the purpose of its actions.

At first sight this type of blind, limited, and automatic behaviour appears to bear little relation to the wider range of human behaviour. It has nevertheless been argued that the original motive force in all human behaviour lies in a specific number of instincts. The fact that man's behaviour is much more adaptable and differs so widely from that of other animals is explained by his superior intelligence which allows him some degree of choice and a capacity to adapt his actions to changing circumstances. In the past many psychologists have attempted to apply the concept of instincts to human behaviour. One of the chief authorities in this field was William McDougall (1933) whose doctrine of instincts had for a time a great impact on psychological thinking. McDougall classified a total of eighteen human instincts which he believed were 'the mainsprings of action.' His list included the gregarious or social instinct, the instincts of fear, sex, assertiveness, disgust, acquisitiveness, and the maternal instinct. Although McDougall was careful to emphasize that the instincts represented only inherited tendencies towards behaviour and not fixed and irrevocable patterns of behaviour, his caution was not maintained by many who later adopted his doctrine of instincts. To say that an aggressive person suffers from an over-developed aggressive (or self-assertive) instinct or that a mother who lacks maternal feeling has an under-developed maternal instinct, is to explain nothing at all. There is also the danger that we begin to think of man's behaviour as being determined by inherited patterns which cannot be altered, thus adopting a static view of behaviour. If a person has an over-developed aggressive instinct we are restricted to diverting his aggressiveness into socially acceptable channels without being able to help him to become a less aggressive person. In recent reading of several British and American books on psychology for nurses I noticed it was commonly stated that people who make good nurses have certain well-developed instincts, such as the maternal or protective instinct, the social instinct, and the instinct of curiosity. It is certainly true that the potential nurse may possess personality traits which especially suit her to her work, but it would be highly misleading to think that such traits were inherited and fixed rather than learned and capable of modification. The doctrine of instincts, in this form, has tended to become part of psychological history and is no longer regarded as a useful aid in understanding human behaviour. Let us consider some of the main criticisms which undermined its validity.

The psychologist, Gordon Allport, questioned the usefulness of the concept of instinctive motivation by his theory of 'functional autonomy' (Allport, 1937). He argued that, although an activity might originate because of an instinctive craving, the activity might itself come in time to yield satisfaction to the individual for its own sake and, in this way, become autonomous or independent from its original source. Thus the adolescent girl may first be stimulated into an interest in her dress and general appearance by the force of the sex instinct. By the time she has reached adulthood, however, she may have developed an interest in dress and appearance which provides its own satisfaction quite in dependent of the original motive. Activities which may have been originated to satisfy an instinct tend to persist generating their own satisfaction and becoming every bit as powerful and demanding as the original need, a fact to which everyone who has tried to stop smoking will testify. If we accept Allport's argument we cannot link every human action with a motivating force which is unlearned and instinctive.

Perhaps the most devastating evidence against the uniformity of human motivation has come from the work of investigators who have studied the behaviour of people in cultures other than our own. These reports showed that many patterns of behaviour which we might tend to think of as being expressions of instincts, and therefore universal, are absent or expressed quite differently in other cultures. The typical maternal behaviour of the mother in our society is, for instance, often regarded as an unlearned activity which is instinctive in origin. It has been shown, however, that in many other cultures there is very little evidence of conventional maternal feelings. In one culture, for instance, children are acquired by the first person who plants a leaf of a tree in front of the house in which a child is born. In other cultures it is the male members of the tribe who rear the baby from infancy and who demonstrate all the attitudes and feelings which we associate with the mother in our culture. Such reports caused a reconsideration of the strength of the maternal instinct in our own culture and it has been shown that it is, indeed, very doubtful whether the mother has any of the inborn tendency to love her child which is implied in the term maternal instinct. Most mothers, in fact, appear to learn gradually to love their child through repeated experience with the child in the first year of life. This sort of argument, of course, does not disprove that there may be some inborn factors in the maternal role. Obviously, for example, there are glandular changes during pregnancy and later which must affect the mother's behaviour. However it does illustrate that, to a large extent, maternal behaviour is influenced and moulded by social custom and that it may vary greatly from one society to another. When evidence for many other so-called instincts laid down by McDougall was looked for in other societies, it was often shown that such evidence was either absent or, again, that the so-called instinctive behaviour was greatly influenced by social factors. Some tribes, for example, show none of the patterns of behaviour which we might associate with an acquisitive instinct. The only two instincts in McDougall's list which appear to be universally present in man's behaviour are the sexual and aggressive instincts. Even here, however, their expression takes on a wide variety of forms from one society to another. Some primitive societies appear to have a minimal amount of aggression in their make-up and are unable to understand such accepted forms of behaviour in our culture as, for example, the waging of organized war. Again, although there are some obvious basic differences in the behaviour of the male relative to the female sex, it is obvious from anthropological evidence that these differences are not nearly so widespread as we regard them in our society. Some primitive societies exist where the males act and generally behave in a manner which we associate with the female role in our culture while the females act in a very masculine way. Even the sex role then is conditioned by social influences. We might conclude from all of this that the work of anthropologists has clearly shown the great influence of the social environment upon the individual's behaviour. In some respects this influence is so powerful as to make it of very doubtful use to speak of any behaviour as being an expression of an inborn instinct. However, in some cases it is equally obvious that, although the social pattern may, to a large extent, decide the particular form of behaviour which will be expressed by the people living in that society, its basic source is still universal and apparently independent of social influences. This is particularly so with McDougall's sexual and aggressive instincts which exist in different forms from society to society but always exist in one form or another.

The instincts of sex and aggression are also the cornerstone of another scheme of instincts put forward by Freud's psychoanalytic school of thought. By reducing the list of instincts to the two fundamental ones of sex and aggression Freud avoided many of the criticisms levelled at McDougall's system. However, it still seems doubtful if all man's complex patterns of behaviour can be ultimately reduced to two instincts, even when the instincts are as fundamental and important as the sexual and aggressive urges. Modern psychoanalytic writers are now accepting that such a view of human behaviour is too restrictive and are giving more attention to conscious activity which is unconnected with the instincts.

The theory of instincts may have proved of little value in its original form but in recent years work has been reported which has revived interest in the subject of instinctive behaviour. This work concentrates upon detailed investigations into the actual mode of operation of instincts in animal behaviour. We have already commented upon the extent to which animals and lower organisms appear to be dominated in their behaviour by instinctive mechanisms which are unlearned and innate. Until recent years there has been no fully adequate way of explaining how these mechanisms actually operate. To take one example, how does it come to be that a bird hatched, born, and reared in isolation from all other birds is still able to respond immediately with panic and flight at the sight of a hawk in the sky? It has had no opportunity of learning in any way from other birds that the hawk is its worst enemy and yet it is able to pick the hawk out from all other birds and respond to it in this way. Is there, then, an inborn knowledge in the bird's mind that the hawk is to be feared?

Recent studies have shown that such activity can be reduced to a simpler pattern which can be experimentally studied. In the case just quoted it has been shown that the bird reacts with panic and flight not to a hawk as such, but to any object which has the same ratio between length of body and wing-span as the hawk. Thus the bird will fly away from two pieces of wood which are erected in such a way. A bird, then, has an inborn tendency to respond to a specific stimulus, in this case a ratio between body size and wing-span. It is suggested that all animals have certain inborn patterns of reaction (termed 'innate release mechanisms') which help the animal to survive and develop. These instinctive reactions are automatic and require no learning but they do require the presence of specific stimuli in the environment to set them functioning. Thus the automatic escape reaction of the bird just mentioned requires the presence of a specific environmental stimulus (in this case the perception of a certain shape in the sky) to trigger it off.

Earlier we referred critically to the so-called maternal instinct in human behaviour. There is, however, no doubt that animals appear to have an inborn capacity to recognize and care for their mother. Ethologists such as Lorenz (1952) have closely studied this response in geese and have demonstrated that the specific stimulus which calls up the instinctive behaviour is, in this case, the visual perception of the first moving object seen after birth. Ordinarily the first moving object seen after birth is, in fact, the mother, but Lorenz has shown that the young will become attached to any other object moving across their field of vision. If, as happened in

Lorenz's work, the first moving object seen is man, the geese will now show all their normal affection for the mother towards man. It has been further demonstrated that there is a specified period during which the instinct will be dormant awaiting the presentation of the correct stimulus which will trigger it off. If, through unusual circumstances, the stimulus is not presented during this period the instinctive apparatus dies off and will not function. Thus, if the bird were isolated from birth, there would be a crucial period of time after which it would have no capacity to react to the sight of the hawk. If released from isolation after this crucial period the bird would probably fall easy prey to the first hawk which appeared. This type of study of animal behaviour is interesting and a fascinating account of it may be found in Lorenz's book *King Solomon's Ring* (Lorenz, 1952).

The reader may reasonably ask, however, what relevance this work has to the study of human behaviour. In recent years psychologists and other workers have successfully applied the new view of instincts to widen our understanding of apparently unlearned responses which appear in the human infant. They have been able to show that such responses as smiling and sucking are innate but also depend for their development upon certain specific environmental stimuli. It might also be argued that, in cases where the appropriate stimuli are absent during the crucial period, the child may develop without one of its normal functions. The response of the child towards the mother, and all this involves, may not be elicited if the appropriate stimulus (the presence of the mother) is missing during the crucial period. This argument would support Bowlby's concept of children who develop an 'affectionless character' following separation from the mother in early infancy although, as we have seen, this concept is by no means verified.

The work of comparative ethologists, such as Lorenz and Tinbergen, has certainly revived interest in the concept of instinctive motivation in human life. Our modern knowledge of the functioning of the brain and nervous system allows us to state a rationale for some of the instincts in earlier classifications and raise them a little above the level of mere description. Thus, McDougall's postulation of an instinct of curiosity receives some support from recent neurophysiological findings which teaches us that the brain requires a constantly changing pattern of stimulation to operate at its most efficient level. Some writers (*e.g.* Fletcher, 1957) have attempted to formulate a new, more comprehensive, theory of instinctive motivation which is a synthesis of the earlier ideas with psycho-analytical theory and ethological findings. Implicit in these modern views is the realization that any system of instinctive motivation must also be concerned with the degree to which the individual's environmental experience may modify his inherited tendencies. In the last section of this part we will consider in more detail this irrevocable link between what is inherited and what is acquired through experience.

Concluding Remarks on Instincts

We have argued here that the formerly held ideas regarding the influence of instincts upon human behaviour are of doubtful value. Man's development depends upon an interplay of two factors, his inherited capacities and the degree to which these capacities are acted upon and shaped by his environmental experiences. The old doctrine of instincts tended to place too great an emphasis upon the innate capacities and under-estimated the extent to which man's personality is affected by social customs and learning from the environment. The new concept of instinct, although more limited, is certainly more scientific in its formulation. In its application to human behaviour it appears to offer a reasonably satisfactory explanation of responses which suddenly appear in infancy without any apparent previous learning. It gives us a link between the behaviour of the animal and that of the human infant. It does not seek to explain the complex patterns of adult behaviour by reducing it to a limited number of instincts and therefore avoids the dangers of the earlier views.

Attitudes

'Opinion is ultimately determined by the feeling and not the intellect' (Herbert Spencer). Of course, much of our adult behaviour is more directly governed by the attitudes and the opinions which we learn and acquire in our experiences throughout life. We have a tendency to believe that when we are faced with any new situation we merely consider all its aspects in a reasonable and rational manner and, thus arrive at an attitude, or an opinion as to how we should act. Our purpose here will be to show that, on the contrary, many of our attitudes and opinions are arrived at, not through the results of careful thinking and deliberation, but are rather motivated by emotions which have little or no reason behind them. The more insight we possess into the origin of our attitudes and the way they affect our behaviour, the more confident we can be that we are masters of our own opinions and actions. Let us first consider some of the ways in which our attitudes, and their expression in our opinions, are formed.

The Development of Attitudes

Firstly, like all other aspects of our personality, our attitudes and opinions may originate within the family group. As children growing up under the influence and guidance of our parents we tend naturally to take over many of their attitudes and opinions. This is most obvious when we look at attitudes and opinions on broad subjects such as politics, religion, etc., where it can be seen that many adults grow up holding the same type of political and religious views as their parents. This is also true, however, of many more personal attitudes such as our moral attitude to right and wrong. If we are brought up, for example, to believe that alcoholic drinking or gambling is a sin, we may find it difficult to change our attitude in later life. Again, to take another example, if we are brought up in a home where it is considered wrong to lose control of one's feelings, we would then tend to be rather intolerant of people who were unable to exert sufficient self-control. Thus we would find it hard to show genuine understanding and sympathy towards a person suffering from a nervous breakdown or a mental illness. Of course, it would be false to assume that we always take over completely the attitudes of our parents on every issue. This may be true to a large extent of the child but, as we have already seen, the adolescent often rebels against the authority of his parents and, at this stage of life, he may adopt attitudes and opinions which are opposite and antagonistic to those of his parents.

The *second* and probably the most obvious way in which we develop our attitudes and opinions is by our uncritical acceptance of the attitudes and opinions of others. Many of our views are coloured and, to a large extent, formed by the opinions of others whom we respect. For example, our opinions on many subjects are taken from what we read in the daily newspapers, what we listen to on the radio, or what we see on the television screen. Of course, we must obtain information in this way if we are going to come to any opinion but the danger is that we often passively accept what we are told in newspapers, books, on the radio, and on television, without even thinking whether our source of information is correct or not. The ideal would be if we could read or in other ways obtain the facts on any subject and then come to our own conclusions. Unfortunately, however, it is often the case that we are given not the facts but someone else's biased opinion on the subject, which we take over without question and soon believe to be our own.

Many of our sources of information are deliberately aimed at engendering certain attitudes of mind and encouraging the recipient to arrive at particular opinions. The whole idea of modern advertising is to foster attitudes by direct and indirect suggestion which will lead the public to act in the ways which suit the advertiser. 'Do you wake in the morning feeling tired, listless, and irritable?' Of course you do, if you are at all human, but already the advertiser has stimulated us into an attitude which will be conducive to his suggestion that the new wonder pills are what we need. Even when we are faced with 'factual' information we cannot afford to accept it uncritically, for facts may easily become fiction when lifted from their context. You may have heard the story of one of our archbishops who was making his first visit to America. On alighting from the plane at New York he was interviewed by newspaper reporters, one of whom asked: 'Will you be going to any night-clubs while in New York?' The archbishop innocently replied: 'Are there any night-clubs here?' The following morning the newspapers showed his photograph with the heading: 'English archbishop's first question on arrival in United States, "Are there any night-clubs here?"' The report was factual but hardly accurate. Obviously life is too short and too complicated for us to be able to study all the facts of every subject before arriving at an opinion. At times we might be better to adopt no opinion at all on a subject rather than accept passively and unquestioningly the opinions of others. This book contains a great deal of verifiable fact, but also, inevitably, a certain amount of personal opinion. The reader may be adopting an unreasonable attitude if he refuses to accept the fact but his attitude will be equally unreasonable if he passively accepts the opinions without first evaluating them on the basis of his own experience.

Even if we had the time and opportunity to collect all the relevant facts on every subject we would be in an impossible position if we had to consider all these facts to reach a conclusion every time we were faced with a new situation. Instead we adopt certain 'frames of reference' upon which we can evaluate and judge any new situation. Thus, membership of a political party or religious group allows us to arrive quickly at opinions on a variety of situations by referring to such a source of authority. It is certainly wrong always to accept the opinions of others but we would not go far in life if we adopted the opposite attitude of always rejecting the views of others. The important point is that we should endeavour to select reliable sources of authority and at the same time, maintain our capacity to arrive at independent conclusions.

Finally we may adopt certain attitudes as an indirect expression of personal problems of which we are not entirely aware. Neurotic and unstable individuals may form certain opinions and adopt certain attitudes mainly to allow them to express their own emotional difficulties. One type of attitude which has been thoroughly investigated is the attitude of intolerance towards people of a different religion, colour, or race than ourselves. These investigations indicated that people who are least tolerant of racial or religious differences are themselves generally emotionally unstable and neurotic. Their intolerant attitude to certain sections of the community allows them to express their own inner insecurity and aggression. Such individuals are, of course, unaware of the true source of their attitudes and opinions which they consider to be founded on rational grounds. There are numerous examples of this function of attitudes apart from racial intolerance. The fear aroused by mental illness, particularly in the less stable members of society, resulted in an aggressive and suspicious attitude towards mental patients which is only now being gradually undone. The passionate feelings aroused by such issues as homosexuality and capital punishment provide further illustrations of the irrational opinions which may be rigidly held when people become emotionally involved.

Effects of Attitudes on Behaviour

Our attitudes to a great extent guide our behaviour. Ideally they should be derived from a personal objective appraisal of the relevant facts of the situation. Unfortunately, as we have seen, many of our attitudes tend to be irrationally developed either through our uncritical acceptance of the opinions of others or as a reflection of our own emotional problems. Reason is adaptable and the more reasonable our attitudes the more we will be able to alter them in the face of contradictory facts. The more our attitudes are founded upon emotion rather than reason, the more rigid they tend to be and the less capable of modification. At times attitudes become so strong, so fixed, and so irrational that we denote them by another term, namely, *prejudices*. A prejudice, then, is an attitude towards any object or situation which is based upon emotion rather than reason and is resistant to contradictory facts. We may, for example, hold the view that all Japanese are cruel and sadistic, this attitude being based upon impressions of the last war. If we visit the country and find that many of the people are kind and considerate in their behaviour, we will reformulate our opinion of the Japanese race to conform with the new facts. If, however, we refuse to alter our views in spite of such contradictory evidence, our attitude must be so irrational and rigid as to be a prejudice. Strong prejudices which are as generalized as that of racial intolerance are, as we have already stated, invariably held by people who are themselves emotionally unbalanced and unstable. There is, however, only a difference of degree between some of our common attitudes and such prejudices. Most of us tend to have our 'blind spots' which lead us to act at times in an irrational manner. Anyone whose work involves the understanding and guidance of others cannot hope to function effectively if blinded by prejudice. Such prejudices control our behaviour and therefore the more insight we possess into the true source of our attitudes the more free we are to direct our actions in a rational manner. The nurse who is prejudiced against certain sets of people on the basis of their colour, religion, or social class, for example, will obviously function less efficiently in her work. The qualities of fair-mindedness and tolerance are essential in nursing or in any other vocation involving interpersonal contact. There is, however, one danger in what we have been saying. Tolerance can sometimes become so exaggerated that it becomes a prejudice in itself. Some people are so determined to be fairminded and to see the pros and cons of every issue that they are unable to come to any decision. In such a case the individual is merely adopting a tolerant attitude as a means of covering up his own indecisiveness. We can respect and tolerate the views of others, accepting that our own outlook will not always be shared by other people, while at the same time feeling free to act according to our personal convictions. Our main aim should be to ensure that our convictions are founded upon logic and not purely upon emotional grounds.

Another psychological term allied to prejudice is that of the *stereotype*. This term describes a generalized and oversimplified belief or opinion which tends to be resistant to contradictory facts. Thus, whereas a prejudice might be thought of as a rigidly extreme attitude, a stereotype refers to a rigidly extreme opinion. Again, forms of stereotyped thinking can be seen in all aspects of human behaviour. The public, for example, tend to have a stereotyped picture of people who suffer from mental illness, which bears little resemblance to the majority of patients. If one shows people around a mental hospital they invariably comment with surprise: 'Why, they look quite normal!' Those concerned with the treatment of the mentally ill often adopt their own stereotypes in categorizing patients by such diagnostic labels as 'schizophrenic,' 'psychopathic,' 'obsessional,' and so on. Such grouping of patients under one heading is, of course, necessary for diagnostic convenience and as a guide to assessing the patient's chance of recovery. If they result, however, in approaching all patients suffering from schizophrenia, for example, in the same way, forgetting that they are distinct individuals with their own problems, then the diagnostic term becomes a stereotype which hinders a true therapeutic understanding. This is equally true of patients whose illness is basically a physical one. If the nurse were to think of her patients simply as 'cases' according to the type of illness involved she would be greatly limiting her usefulness to the patient. Most stereotypes develop as generalizations of opinions formed out of our too limited past experience. If we are to form any opinions we must, of course, generalize on the basis of our experience. Such opinions only become stereotypes when they are rigidly held and are not changed to fit in with later experiences.

An interesting and worrying illustration of the influence of diagnostic stereotyping is provided by Rosenhan's (1973) study. He rehearsed a number of normal adults to attend psychiatric out-patient clinics, feigning the symptom of hearing voices. Each of these pseudo-patients were admitted to hospital with the possible diagnosis of schizophrenia. After admission they behaved normally and were finally discharged after about three weeks as 'remitted schizophrenics'.

However, the most interesting findings in the study related to what Rosenhan terms 'the stickinesses of the diagnostic label . In a series of vivid examples he demonstrates how the diagnostic label of schizophrenia causes hospital staff to relate to the pseudo-patients as if they were sub-human aliens. Sensible questions put by the patients to the staff were often ignored or answered in oblique ways. Female nursing staff adjusted their underclothing in full view of male patients, as if the patients were non-existent. A pseudo-patient who kept a daily diary was described as a 'compulsive note-taker'. Another who was usually first in the meal line-up was described as having 'oral fixation problems', and yet another was thought to be hallucinating simply because he sat looking out of the ward window. The point that Rosenhan makes is that, once diagnosed as psychotic, every behaviour emitted by the individual is seen as reflecting his diagnostic label. It is literally impossible to be seen as sane in insane places. The fact that the hospitals concerned in this study represented a reasonable cross-section of U.S.A. institutions and that the staff were well trained professionals who cared for their patients does not offer much cheer. It would seem that it is lamentably easy for even the most humane hospital professional to unwittingly begin to substitute a diagnostic stereotype for the individual personality of the patient.

Concluding Remarks on Attitudes

We might conclude that even a cursory study of the attitudes and opinions which motivate human behaviour suggests that man is not the creature of reason that we sometimes suppose him to be. Our adult attitudes tend to be greatly influenced by our family background and by the social context to which we belong. At the same time we must remember that man is not passively moulded by these social influences. They stimulate him to respond selectively in his own unique way in terms of his own pattern of resources. Some of our attitudes tend to be particularly 'egocentric' and largely immune from social influences in that they represent inner problems of which we have limited insight. When such conditions are extreme our attitudes become prejudices, our opinions become stereotypes, and we surrender to some degree our capacity to control our own destiny. People tend to be carried along upon the wave of their prejudices, understanding little of what lies beneath the surface of their own feelings. If our attitudes and opinions are flexible and controlled by reason they allow us to organize our behaviour in an economic and efficient manner. If, however, they become rigid and emotionally controlled they result in a restriction of our personality and operate as a barrier to true self expression.

During her training the nurse must cultivate certain attitudes towards her work. These will include a sense of responsibility, pride in herself, and in what she does and an attitude of tolerance and respect for people in general. She must guard against attitudes and opinions which, although perhaps held by others, will make her less effective in her work. Her professional and personal standards must be high for not only does her work call for skilled devotion but she also functions as a symbol of reliability and integrity to others. The more she can be aware of, and in control of, her own motives the easier will be her task.

Emotions

In the preceding section it was suggested that many of our attitudes, opinions and actions are emotionally determined. Emotions are indeed such an integral part of being human that it is difficult to contemplate what life might be like without the warmth and colour they bring to our experiences. Perhaps the French philosopher Descartes' dictum 'I think therefore I am' could be just as convincingly restated as 'I *feel* therefore I am'. Feelings constitute one of the most private areas of human experience and are therefore notoriously difficult to examine. We can express our thoughts adequately in words but feelings are much more difficult to communicate, tending to lose much of their true flavour in the translation. If someone tells us that he feels joyful or anxious we may infer that he is experiencing the same inner state we ourselves have experienced when joyful or anxious. However, we have no very secure grounds for assuming such an identity of feelings and their verbal symbols. An alternative indication is given by the facial expressions and other actual physical signs which may be observed by a person reacting emotionally. If observers are shown filmed excerpts of people in emotionally arousing situations they are usually able to agree on whether the person in the film is angry, frightened, happy etc. However, if the film depicts only the person and does not give any information as to the situation which is stimulating him, then observers often find it difficult to identify the emotion being experienced. Another complicating factor here is that emotions may be expressed in different ways in different cultures. However, emotions involve not only changes in facial expression or outer appearance but also internal changes in the autonomic and central nervous system. More recently psychologists have attempted to measure these internal reactions in the hope that these may provide more reliable indices of emotional activity. Before examining the outcome of such attempts to apply the objective scientific approach to the measurement of emotional reactions we shall first consider how emotions appear to develop and differentiate in early life.

The Development of Emotions

There would seem to be little doubt that, like most human responses, many of our emotional reactions are learned through repeated interplay with our environment. In other words, some situations make us happy, sad, frightened, angry or disgusted because of our earlier experiences with similar situations. However, it is quite possible that some of our basic emotions are innate rather than learned and will tend to occur in certain situations regardless of previous experience. Most careful studies of the emotional responses of infants and young children suggest that our range of emotional responses initially is very limited and develops slowly in a fairly uniform order during childhood. Earlier observations (*e.g.* Watson, 1919) of infants led psychologists to conclude that the three basic unlearned emotions were fear, rage and love and that these were evident from birth. Later work indicated that it was the adult observer who tended to 'read in' these emotions from the infants' reactions to situations and that it was impossible to reliably differentiate any specific emotions in early infancy. At the same time, it is clearly evident that young infants do display some undifferentiated form of emotion for which the most appropriate term would appear to be 'excitement'. Systematic longitudinal studies (*e.g.* Bridges, 1931) suggest that somewhere around the third month of life this emotional excitement differentiates into the two opposite emotions of delight and distress. Later these emotions are in

Figure 2

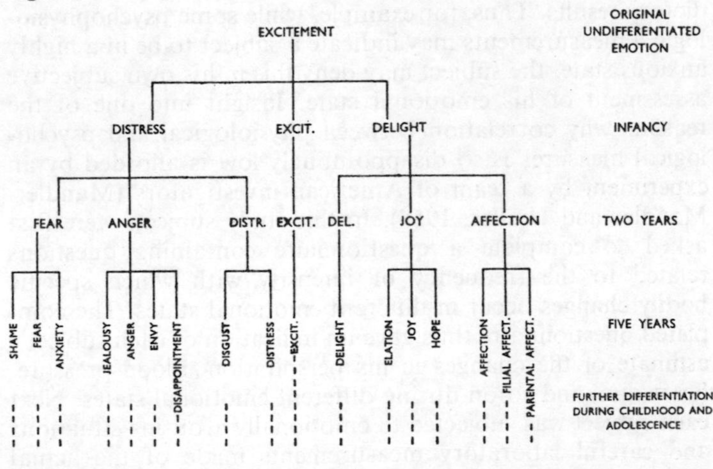

Emotional development in childhood.

turn further partitioned, that of delight dividing up into the more specific emotions of joy and affection, while emotions of fear, disgust and anger develop from the cruder emotion of distress. A schematic representation of this view of emotional development is shown in Figure 2 on previous page.

The Measurement of Emotions

As we have already seen, there are perhaps three main approaches to measuring emotional changes. We may ask people to describe their emotions, or observe their behaviour in emotionally arousing situations, or measure the internal bodily changes which occur during an emotional experience. Psychologists have devised many different types of questionnaires and rating scales in which subjects' responses are collated to provide quantitative measurements of such emotional reactions as anxiety, anger and depression. Investigators have also made systematic observations of individual reactions to different types of stressful situations. Other studies have led to the development of many techniques designed to measure some of the complex physiological components of emotional experience. Thus, the changes in such functions as heart rate, pulse rate, blood pressure, breathing activity, and in the electrical resistance of the skin have all been utilized in the search for objective correlates of emotion. An allied approach has involved the biochemical analysis of the changes in glandular secretions occurring during emotional change.

Unfortunately, these different approaches often yield contradictory results. Thus, for example, while some psychophysiological measurements may indicate a subject to be in a highly anxious state, the subject may deny this in his own subjective assessment of his emotional state. Insight into one of the reasons why correlation between physiological and psychological measures is so disappointingly low is afforded by an experiment by a team of American investigators (Mandler, Mandler and Uviller, 1958). In this study subjects were first asked to complete a questionnaire containing questions related to the frequency of intensity with which specific bodily changes occur in different emotional states. The completed questionnaire thus gave an indication of each subject's estimate of the changes in his perspiration, blood pressure, heart rate, and so on during different emotional states. Next each subject was subjected to emotionally arousing situations and careful laboratory measurements made of the actual changes in these various bodily changes. A comparison of the two measurements demonstrated that those subjects who had rated themselves as experiencing intense bodily changes tended to overestimate the actual changes which occurred, while low raters tended to underestimate the frequency and intensity of internal emotional changes. These results help to explain why psychological and physiological measurements of emotion are seldom in complete agreement with each other.

A similar lack of success has been evident in the attempts of psychologists to distinguish the specific patterns of bodily changes accompanying specific emotions. Thus the physiological changes occurring in the separate emotions of say anger and fear overlap to such an extent as to make it extremely difficult to differentiate between them, purely on the evidence of the physiological measures. A likely explanation of this inability to identify specific emotional patterns is suggested in an interesting experiment by Schachter and Singer (1962). In this study three groups of subjects were given injections of adrenalin but each group was given a different set of instructions. One group was informed what effects might be expected to occur, another was misinformed (led to expect the wrong changes) and the third was left completely ignorant as to the possible effects of the injection. A fourth group was injected with a saline solution and given no instructions. Unknown to the rest of the subjects the experimenters had 'planted' some subjects in each group with instructions to simulate either the emotion of anger or that of elation. The results clearly demonstrated that the subjects who showed the most intense emotional reactions of anger or elation were those who had been given adrenalin but either misinformed, or left ignorant of its likely effects. These findings support the view that although the internal physiological changes cause a heightening of generalized emotional arousal, the specific emotion experienced depends greatly upon the person's interpretation of the situation.

If this view is correct we are unlikely to find a specific pattern of physiological change corresponding to each emotion we experience. All emotions might instead share a common pattern of physiological changes. If, for example, we are threatened this situation will induce a heightened level of generalized emotional arousal which may be experienced by us as anger or fear, depending upon how we perceive the situation. Our final emotional experience is thus seen to be an amalgum of both affective and cognitive factors, the former providing the intensity of the experience and the latter deciding its quality.

This way of looking at the emotions has led psychologists to take an increasing interest in individual differences in the *duration* and *intensity* of emotional reactions. Everyday observation suggests that people vary greatly in the strength of their emotional reactions. Some people appear to have a lower threshold of emotionality which causes them to react intensely and for a longer time to situations which evoke little or no reaction from others. There are some suggestions that such individual differences reflect differences in the level of activity of the autonomic nervous system which may be inherited or constitutional in origin. Research studies have demonstrated clear differences in the autonomic re-activity of young infants (Richmond and Lustman, 1955) and even in neonates (Mirsky, 1958). Pronounced individual differences in the autonomic re-activity of adult subjects have also been demonstrated (Lacey, Bateman and Van Lehn, 1953). Furthermore, evidence has been produced to support the view that some individuals show fairly specific forms of autonomic re-activity which render them particularly vulnerable to stress diseases. Thus neurotic patients have been shown to have an elevated blood pressure response to stressful situations compared to normal control subjects (Malmo and Shagass, 1952). Patients with cardiovascular symptoms show an abnormally high cardiovascular response to stress while patients with headache complaints respond to the same type of stress with increases in muscle tension. There is then good reason to suppose that the autonomically overactive person is more likely to develop certain patterns of symptoms as a result of repeated exposure to stressful situations. It is worth reminding ourselves here that this picture of the high autonomic reacter does not necessarily coincide with the picture we have in mind when we think of an 'overemotional' person. Two people might have the same tendency to have intense and prolonged autonomic responses when angered but differ greatly in the manner in which these autonomic changes are discharged in behaviour. One might habitually 'blow-up' in a direct expression of rage while the other may be the type of person who finds it difficult to express his hostility. Consideration of such individual differences in autonomic reactivity leads us naturally to that area of common ground between the physician and the psychiatrist—psychosomatic medicine.

Psychosomatic Disorders

The term *psychosomatic* (formed from the Greek words 'psyche' meaning mind and 'soma' meaning body) has been employed to embrace a number of disorders which, although involving pathological bodily changes, are thought to be partly a result of psychological stress. At times this diagnostic category has been applied so loosely to such a wide variety of disorders that it has functioned as a temporary waste-bin for conditions whose physical aetiology is at the time unclear. Thus, for example, certain types of eye infections were at one time regarded as psychosomatic, the recurrent watering of the eyes being interpreted as 'repressed weeping' due to unconscious depression. As soon as it was realized that these conditions were caused by a transfer of infection from the hands when rubbing the eyes the psychosomatic label was withdrawn and these contact infections regarded as physical in origin.

However, there are a number of disorders to which the term psychosomatic can be applied with some justification. One of the most noticeable bodily changes accompanying excessive emotion is a change in the normal breathing rhythm. This combined with the known influence of the parasympathetic nerves in contracting the musculature of the bronchial tubes has led to such respiratory conditions as *asthma* being regarded as a psychosomatic illness. This view has stimulated a wealth of research studies on the family background of asthmatic children which certainly seem to agree that these children are more anxious, insecure and over dependent than non-asthmatics. Some reports of the pattern of asthmatic attacks shown by individual patients offer very convincing evidence of psychological precipitants. Thus, for example, Metcalfe (1956) plotted the asthmatic attacks of a young married woman and was able to demonstrate that almost 90 per cent of these attacks immediately followed the patient's visits to her mother's home. However, even if a relationship can be established between asthma and specific personality factors this does not allow us to assume that these factors *cause* the asthma. It may well be that any chronic condition such as asthma, which is both frightening to the child and limits his activity, produces personality changes as a *reaction* to the illness. Indeed, other research studies have already established that children with any chronic physical handicap are more likely to become insecure and anxious and be over-protected by their well meaning parents.

As an increase in blood pressure is a common response to stress it might be thought that *essential* hypertension could develop as a result of continual psychological trauma. A number of investigations of hypertensive and non-hypertensive patients have confirmed that whereas the blood pressure level of the latter group falls quickly when the stress is removed, that of hypertensive patients shows a prolonged elevation. Studies of the personalities of hypertensive individuals illustrate the role of aggressive impulses in the development of a chronic hypertensive state. The findings of most of these studies suggest that the hypertensive patient is not necessarily an abnormally aggressive individual but rather a person who, as a result of circumstances and his own inhibitions, has found himself repeatedly unable to discharge his anger.

However, probably the most frequent and certainly the best demonstrated of the psychosomatic disorders are the digestive disorders such as *peptic ulcer*. One of the classical demonstrations of the effects of continual changes on gastric functions was provided by Wolf and Wolff's (1947) study of one patient. As a boy this patient had performed on him an uncompleted gastrostomy which left him with a gastric fistula through which he fed himself with pre-masticated food. Later in life this patient's unusual physical state allowed investigators to directly observe the effect of natural and artificially induced stress on his gastric functions. When the patient was thwarted and made angry his mucous membrane became congested and red and there was a noticeable increase in his acid secretion. In contrast a depressive mood caused the membrane to become pale and led to a drastic reduction in acid secretion. When his gastric mucus could no longer offer sufficient protection to the membrane the increased acid secretion caused ulceration.

This rather unique case offers a striking illustration of the possible relationship between emotional changes and ulcer formation. It is a common belief that some individuals are more 'ulcer-prone' through their holding down of jobs involving much responsibility and stress. However, many people who are exposed to great stress and responsibility in everyday life never develop ulcers. There is considerable evidence that ulcer patients tend to secrete much more acid in their stomach than non-ulcer patients. Some research has demonstrated that ulcer-prone individuals may be predicted by prior measures of their stomach secretions. Thus in one experiment large numbers of American servicemen were examined and those with very high and very low levels of secretory activity extracted. When these two groups were reassessed at the end of their military training only individuals in the high secretory group had developed ulcers. Similar results were found in civilian populations. It has also been demonstrated that high secretory activity in neonates is directly related to high secretory levels in the parents (Mirsky, 1958). While such work suggests the possibility that some people are constitutionally predisposed to develop ulcers because of their autonomic activity, once again the individual personality appears to be an important contributing factor. For instance, in the study just mentioned (Weiner, Thaler, Reiser and Mirsky, 1957) those who developed peptic ulcers not only had high secretory levels but had pronounced difficulty in expressing their aggressive feelings.

It is interesting to reflect that ulcer victims and others more vulnerable to the stresses of everyday life are often advised as to the therapeutic gains of a good night's restful sleep. However, careful studies of the body's activity during sleep tend to contradict the assumption that in sleep we enjoy a temporary respite from stress. Observations of ulcer patients demonstrate that during R.E.M. sleep when we are dreaming (see Ch. 8), heavy secretions of stomach acids occur. Indeed, it would seem that we are at least as vulnerable to stress when we are asleep as when we are awake.

Psychosomatic medicine is a very wide topic which has been treated briefly and superficially in the foregoing discussion. However, it would seem that all psychosomatic disorders probably involve two interacting causal factors—the personality of the individual and his constitutional predisposition. Modern treatment of most of these conditions consists of combining medical treatment for the physical symptoms with psychological treatment to alleviate the stress which helps to produce the symptoms.

Concluding Remarks on Emotions

Although much of our normal and abnormal behaviour is determined by our feelings, the affective side of human experience has been explored with less success than many other areas of psychological investigation. One of the main problems is that our feelings are highly personal and subjective experiences which are difficult to communicate and almost impossible to study objectively. While attempts to accurately measure the physiological components of emotion have had some success in producing more reliable assessments, their validity is often in question. Most of us are acquainted with the interesting studies of Masters and Johnson (1966) on human sexual activities. In these studies a number of volunteers indulged in sexual intercourse and masturbation while a multitude of ingenious instruments recorded their physical and emotional changes. Although reports of this research upset many people, there is no doubt that the study was conducted with excessive ethical precautions and with full scientific rigour. It provided a great deal of extremely useful information about normal and abnormal sexual functioning which acted as a welcome palliative to some of the uninformed nonsense written around this subject in the past. However, it is very doubtful whether this study provides any valid information regarding the emotional changes which occur in this most private of all human activities. Some areas of human experience are so intrinsically private and subjective as to defeat all attempts at scientific measurement. Long may this state endure!

QUESTIONS

1. What objections might be put forward to the view that human behaviour is fundamentally governed by innate instincts?

2. Discuss the ways in which our attitudes and opinions develop. To what extent do they guide our adult behaviour?

3. Discuss the type of attitudes which the nurse must try to develop, and comment on the need for her to prevent her thinking being unduly influenced by stereotypes and prejudices.

4. To what extent can our emotional state affect our physical well-being?

6. Unconscious Motivation

The Concept of the 'Unconscious'

By unconscious motivation we refer to the fact that many of the factors which influence and motivate our behaviour are outside our awareness and are in this sense unconscious. However, this distinction loses much of its strength when we remember that even our conscious attitudes and opinions may be influenced by factors which are outside our field of awareness. In other words, we have already recognized that we are not always fully aware of the causes behind our own actions. At one time it was thought that we could only be affected in our behaviour by experiences of which we had been aware. In recent years, however, we have come to realize that this is not the case. When we are concentrating on something we may be unaware of other things going on outside our immediate field of attention. It can be easily demonstrated, however, that we may at the same time be taking in these extraneous stimuli without being consciously aware of this process. Let us take two illustrations of this type of perception in operation. The first example comes from the subject of intelligence testing which we will be discussing later. It is a known fact that some people who give intelligence tests always tend to obtain a higher level of performance from the people tested than is the case with other testers. Sometimes this is caused by the tester. without being aware of it, giving valuable aids and hints to the person doing the test who, himself, is often unaware that he is being guided by these hints. For instance, it is difficult for the examiner to avoid slight changes in his facial expression when he sees the subject about to point to the wrong solution. The tester's change of expression may give a hint to the person being tested that he is on the wrong track and thus enable him eventually to arrive at the right solution. Or, conversely, any indication of pleasure on the face of the tester may give the person being tested a hint that he is now on the right track. The important aspect of this situation is that very often both the tester and the person being tested are unaware that they have given out or taken up these slight hints or 'cues' as they are called.

A second example of the same principle is taken from the field of modern advertising. Normally advertisements are presented to us visually and we are at liberty to evaluate the suggestion of the advertiser critically and perhaps reject it. It has now been demonstrated that a verbal or pictorial advertisement, which is presented in such a way as to make it impossible for us to perceive it consciously, still affects our behaviour. An experiment has been tried out in cinemas in which a short caption urging the audience to buy ice cream was flashed across the screen with such a rapid rate of exposure that the audience were not even aware of its existence. Although the audience had not been conscious of the advertisement the proof of its effectiveness lay in the fact that, during the experiment, ice cream sales increased by a highly significant amount. Many more examples of this sort of thing can be quoted, all of them indicating that our perceptions, our thinking, and our behaviour may often be affected by what we call *subliminal cues*. The word subliminal is used here to denote the fact that these stimuli or cues are received below the threshold of our conscious awareness and thus mean that their effects on our behaviour are unconscious. Most people do not have any great difficulty in accepting such facts and, of course, they can be experimentally demonstrated quite easily. Many people who would accept this, however, have great difficulty in accepting the psycho-analytic concept of unconscious motivation although the two are nevertheless connected. Freud, who founded the psycho-analytic school of thinking, showed that there was a part of our mind which he termed the unconscious which contained thoughts, wishes, feelings, and ideas which were outside the range of our conscious awareness. Freud also showed that many of the thoughts and impulses in the unconscious had at one time been conscious but had been 'repressed,' or pushed out, of our conscious mind into the unconscious. These impulses which were repressed in this way are usually of an unpleasant nature. For example, the young child has a great love for his parents but at times they interfere with things which he wishes to do and, if this interference is too pronounced, the child feels hostility towards his parents. Having such hostile ideas towards the loved parents on whom he is dependent makes him feel guilty and afraid of the consequences which would follow the expression of his hostile impulses. He solves this situation by 'repressing' his hostile feelings out of his conscious mind. However, although they are no longer conscious they are still as it were at the back of his mind, in the part of the mind which Freud called the unconscious. It is perhaps easiest to regard the mind as being divided into two portions—the conscious and the unconscious—with a barrier between the two. In certain situations, for example in dreaming, this barrier is weakened and the impulses, wishes, and ideas in the unconscious flow over into the conscious part of the mind. Often these ideas and impulses are so foreign to our conscious thinking and so unpleasant that they become conscious, even in sleep, only in a disguised and distorted form. This accounts for the fact that our dreams often appear nonsensical and meaningless. Freud also differentiated between what he termed the 'Preconscious,' which contained ideas just outside of our conscious awareness, and the 'Unconscious' proper which contained more powerful but inaccessible feelings. The material in our preconscious could be made conscious by directing our attention on to it but unconscious material could not be so easily elicited. Subliminal cues of the type to which we referred would probably be thought of by psychoanalysts as belonging to the preconscious part of the mind.

Although this dividing of the mind into the separate compartments of Conscious, Preconscious, and Unconscious is a useful and convenient aid to our thinking it is obviously not to be taken too literally. There seems no reason to suppose that there is a separate region in the brain structurally demarcated as the unconscious. Other psychologists such as Piaget (1951) object to the sharp distinction between consciousness and unconsciousness, preferring to think in terms of different levels of consciousness, the lowest of which are normally inaccessible to conscious reflection. Normally adult man has a fair measure of insight into his own motives in that he has the capacity of reflecting upon the reasons for his behaviour. When emotionally or neurotically disturbed, however, this capacity for reflection is lowered and he is less able to become aware of the motives which dictate his behaviour. In this sense the neurotic person is less able effectively to control his actions which are directed by impulses of which he is unaware. In cases of severe mental illness the psychotic patient's conduct is wholly dominated by impulses of which he has no control and no insight. By losing his capacity to reflect upon his own actions he loses his hold on reality. The aim of psychological treatment of mental disorder is to aid the patient in recovering control of his own actions by helping him to become aware of the nature of the unconscious motives which are controlling him.

When Freud first outlined his concept of the unconscious he used psychological language and terminology in describing the dynamics of the mind. He himself looked forward to the day when his metaphysical system could be complemented by an increase in our understanding of the actual physiological mechanisms involved in thinking. Although we are still very far from achieving this goal advances in recent years have, probably for the first time, brought this possibility at least on to the horizon. We know, from previous work and from common experience, that our sense organs are being constantly bombarded by a great variety of sensory stimuli from the environment. If we record a conversation on a tape recorder we are often surprised, when playing it back, to discover a number of distracting noises which have also been recorded at the same time as the conversation. These noises may include the sound of passing traffic, the ticking of a clock, footsteps in a passageway and so on, and they detract from our ability to concentrate on the play-back of the recorded conversation. At the time of the conversation, however, we were probably unaware of these distractions and had no difficulty in focusing our attention on the conversation in hand. In other words, we have some means at our disposal which allows us to selectively narrow our attention when concentration is necessary by suppressing from our awareness simultaneous events which would otherwise be distracting. The example of the tape recorder illustrates this for only one sensory channel, but at any moment of time our senses are being subjected to stimuli, not only through the ear but through all other sense organs as well. Such diverse stimulation is picked up by our sense organs but, particularly when we are concentrating on one thing, the extraneous stimuli do not appear to register in the brain as part of our span of awareness. To put this another way, it would appear that, during the attentive state, our nervous system is able to monitor for us the information coming in through the sense organs so that information irrelevant to the task in hand is inhibited.

While our conscious thinking is, on the whole, rational, logical, and adapted to reality, our unconscious thinking is irrational, emotionally determined, and egocentric. The type of thinking which dominates the behaviour of the mentally disturbed may in fact be compared to the type of thinking which, as we have already discussed, is typical of childhood.

If the mental disturbance is extreme the patient's thinking becomes so primitive as to be comparable with the very young child who confuses his own inner thoughts with outer events. In this state he loses touch with reality and loses control over his own behaviour. Like the child he only has to think about something to imagine that the event has actually occurred. He may interpret his own thoughts as 'voices' coming from the world outside him or he may believe that his own visual images are 'real' events occurring in the external world.

We do not need, however, to limit ourselves to mental illness to obtain evidence of the workings of the unconscious mental activity. The state of dreaming has already been cited as a situation where normal man loses touch with reality. As we become drowsy we gradually renounce control over the direction of our thoughts which begin to follow a strange illogical pattern. As our level of consciousness is further lowered we confuse our internal images with external events so that we can no longer clearly distinguish between what is 'real' and what is 'imaginary'. Finally, in the full state of sleep, our dream thinking takes an irrational and bizarre form as we relapse into a world of fantasy where logic no longer applies.

In our every-day life, however, we find many examples of our unconscious wishes and feelings breaking through to become evident in our behaviour. Many common every-day 'slips of the tongue' can be explained in this way. Some time ago a patient who was leaving hospital insisted on giving me her Edinburgh address in case I should ever be able to visit her. I thought it a little strange as I knew enough of the situation to be fairly sure that the patient's feelings towards me were anything but positive. My opinion was soon verified as the patient dictated 'in error' the address of a friend in Cornwall. While being consciously polite she was unconsciously showing her desire to place as much distance between us as possible. Another personal example of a similar 'slip' occurred very recently when I was writing to a colleague working in another psychological department. Instead of addressing my letter to 'The Department of Clinical Psychology,' I 'mistakenly' addressed the envelope to 'The Department of Cynical Psychology,' an 'error' which my colleague was quick to interpret. Many of you will have been amused by similar slips in newspapers which often betray the writer's or the printer's true feelings. My favourite here is the English newspaper which printed the following notice: 'In the article on the local police in our last edition we inadvertently referred to our "Defective Police Force". We apologize for this error which, of course, should have read "Detective Police Farce".'

Earlier we commented on the view that human beings could not achieve happiness without a great deal of self deception. We answered this view by saying that the mature adult had no need to deceive himself. In so far as he has insight into his own limitations and capabilities he is able to look in the mirror at his true reflection. This, however, is a rather idealistic view and it is a sad truth that most of us look only in a mirror which reflects an image of ourselves as we would like to be, rather than as we actually are. Most of us have impulses and wishes which we would rather not admit to ourselves and to others. Many of these unacceptable feelings lie outside our normal awareness but threaten to invade and influence our behaviour at any time. We ward off these unacceptable urges by a variety of manoeuvres, some of which have come to be known as Personality Defence Mechanisms. These personality defence mechanisms are ways of disguising our unconscious impulses which reach consciousness during the wakened state. It is important to remember that these mechanisms allow us not only to mislead other people as to our real feelings, but also allow us to mislead ourselves in so far as they conceal from our conscious awareness aspects of our personality which we do not wish to recognize. Examples of these mechanisms at work can be seen in the behaviour of the mentally ill, but, as we shall show, every individual makes use of such mechanisms constantly in one form or another to protect their personality and to bolster their self-esteem.

Personality Defence Mechanisms

1. Repression

We may define repression as a process by which we bar unacceptable impulses, feelings, or thoughts from consciousness. Indirect references have already been made to this process at work in every-day life. Many of the things we 'forget' would be better described as being repressed in that we avoid unpleasant consequences by removing the memory from our conscious mind. Only too often we forget the unpleasant experiences we have had while retaining a conscious memory of the more pleasant experiences. Ask any adult about their childhood and they will usually say that it was a very happy one. They will have little difficulty in reviving memories of enjoyable experiences but will run up against a defensive wall of repression in respect of unpleasant past experiences which at the time caused them concern. Like most things human beings do, forgetting is an active process which usually serves some personal purpose. Some time ago I had an argument with a colleague during which I said something which, unknown to me, both hurt and annoyed my friend. A few days later I asked to borrow a book which he had at home. Although he prided himself upon an excellent memory he nevertheless forgot to bring the book on three consecutive mornings. Annoyed at his 'forgetfulness' my friend put the book into his brief-case as soon as he arrived home on the fourth evening. This precaution was, however, of little avail for he arrived at work the following morning without his brief-case, an omission which had never happened before. By this time he decided that there were factors in the situation other than carelessness and we jokingly sat down to discuss the possible reasons for his lapses of memory. Before we knew it our conversation had turned to our argument of a few days previous and this time he showed his annoyance at my earlier remarks. I was able to correct the impression I had given him and convince him that no personal slight had been intended. The following morning he brought in the book. A similar explanation is often applicable when we forget appointments with people whom we dislike or to whom we feel hostile.

More severe and disabling effects of repression can be seen in many neurotic states. For example, during the last war many soldiers suffered hysterical illnesses which were motivated by their repression of some very terrifying experience which they had suffered during battle. In these cases treatment often consists of the individual being aided to re-live the buried memory or the terrifying experience and to work off his feelings of anxiety. Some cases of loss of memory or amnesia can be similarly explained in terms of repression as, for instance, the unhappily married man who has a loss of memory covering the whole period of his marriage. It is important to remember that, in repression, the actual memory of the event may be retained, while the feelings associated with the event may become unconscious. Some neurotic patients have a full and vivid memory of experiences in childhood which caused them great anxiety but have completely repressed all the terror associated with the experience. Repression seldom works completely effectively. Although the memory or the feeling associated with it may be displaced from our conscious awareness it usually continues to exert some effect upon our behaviour. This effect may take the form of a vague uneasiness or, in more extreme cases, the appearance of neurotic symptoms. We need not look far for examples of repression in the behaviour of patients in hospital. Only too often does the patient conveniently 'forget' to come for that examination or to take that unpleasant treatment.

2. Projection

Projection may be defined as a complete denial of our own unconscious impulses which produce tension by the attribution of these impulses to some external object or person. This process can be seen to operate in many ever-day situations. To take one example, we might cite the case of the husband who has the desire to be unfaithful to his wife but, instead of accepting consciously these desires, projects them on to his wife whom he accuses of infidelity. Probably the most obvious example of projection is the picture of the old maid who imagines that she is being followed by men who wish to make advances to her. An extreme case of projection can be seen in the case of the paranoid patient who projects his own aggressive feelings on to others, causing him to believe that others are persecuting him and meaning him harm.

In many cases what is projected is the blame for any situation which, for some reason, the individual is unable to accept. Some people are never able to accept their share of responsibility, instead habitually projecting it on to others. The person who presents a consistent pattern of this type in his behaviour is described as having an *extra-punitive* attitude. (The opposite extreme is represented by the *intro-punitive* person who repeatedly blames himself for any failure regardless of the circumstances.)

We have all met people who, rather than accept their own inadequacies, project them on to their surroundings. The young nurse, feeling unsure of herself, may project her insecurity on to the hospital and its staff, blaming circumstances for her lack of progress. The unco-operative patient may project his resistance on to the hospital staff and feel that the nurses are deliberately setting out to annoy him.

3. Introjection and Identification

The process of introjection operates in an opposite way to that of projection. Here the individual incorporates within his own personality aspects of external objects or persons. We have already referred to the way in which the child introjects the attitudes and opinions of the parents so that these become part of his own personality. As adults we tend to introject aspects of our environment so that they become an integral part of our lives. The dedicated nurse extends the range of her own personality by incorporating the ideals and principles of nursing during her training. Thereafter she will be affected personally by any events which affect the profession as a whole. Identification is a somewhat similar mechanism which, however, operates temporarily and does not so radically alter the personality as does introjection. We have already referred to this process in our earlier discussion on the child's identification with parents and the adolescent's tendency to model himself on new figures. Identification, in fact, plays a primary part in all learning in that what we learn in any situation depends as much upon the personality of the teacher as the material to be learned. Perhaps the most obvious illustration of identification in nursing lies in the young student nurse's inclination to model herself upon those under whom she trains. Earlier we commented on the capacity of the nurse to identify herself with her patients as a necessary quality of effective nursing. In some senses both introjection and identification may be viewed as processes which aid the individual in her development and in relating herself to her environment. It is only when these processes become extreme that they have the opposite effect of limiting individual development. Thus the intro-punitive attitude is essentially an extreme form of introjection while extreme identification might cause the nurse to take upon herself her patients' problems and symptoms. Some people do show in their behaviour an over-readiness to introject the views of others and to identify themselves so completely with others as to have little personality of their own. They function not as independent persons but as shadows or echoes of the personalities of others.

4. Displacement

Displacement may be defined as the redirection of feelings from their source on to a substitute object. Displacement can have two main functions. It can allow the individual to obtain some release of repressed feelings by displacing these feelings on to another object or person. The adolescent who represses his hostile feelings towards his own father may find a substitute outlet for his feelings in acting aggressively towards other figures in authority, such as his teacher. Displacement, however, need not always be confined to repressed feelings. It may function as a means of satisfying feelings which, because of circumstances, can no longer be expressed. Thus, the mother whose children are now grown up and married may find a new expression of her maternal feelings by displacing these on to a domestic pet such as a dog or budgie. A special form of displacement occurs in psycho-analysis when the patient displaces feelings originally felt towards parents and others on to the analyst. This form of displacement, known as *the transference*, operates to some extent in every intimate human relationship. Our approach to every new situation is coloured by our past experiences. The adult patient's reactions to illness usually contain some transference of feelings from previous illnesses in childhood. His feelings towards the doctor, the nurse, and the hospital will be influenced by feelings aroused by similar experiences in the past. The nurses's attitude to her patients will in turn contain some elements transferred from her earlier relations with important people in her life. This, of course, is merely another way of saying that a person's reactions to any present situation will be greatly influenced by their previous experiences and that therefore no human situation can be assessed accurately if only the present circumstances are taken into account.

Much of the otherwise puzzling behaviour of patients in the wards of mental hospitals becomes understandable if viewed in terms of displacement. The feelings of disordered patients towards others often take the form of extreme liking or extreme hostility. Many of them become excessively attached to their nurses, the extent of their attachment being itself influenced by the type of transference of which we have spoken. In her daily work coping with a large number of patients, the nurse often unwittingly incurs the wrath of a patient who may resent her attention to other patients in the ward. Because of his positive attachment to the nurse the patient is unable to rid himself of the aggression by making a direct attack upon the nurse. Instead he may find a substitute outlet for his feelings by attacking another patient or even by breaking windows. In such cases the patient's disturbed behaviour can only be controlled by an awareness of the true source of the disturbance. In the general hospital the opposite type of situation is more likely to arise when the patient displaces his annoyance at being ill, or his anxiety regarding his family's welfare, in the form of awkward and unco-operative behaviour towards the nursing staff. The displacement of feelings is, of course, not a prerogative of the patient. The nurse may act out on her patients her ill temper which has been aroused by some personal situation. One can easily imagine a train of events and consequences set into motion through, let us say, the doctor having a row with his wife before coming on duty. During the ward round he vents his anger on the ward sister by being over-critical and abusive. The sister is upset by this experience and, in turn, displaces her anger on to her nurses who finally transmit it to the patients. Some patients become upset by the abrupt manner of the nurses and, in no time at all, we have a disturbed and unhappy ward left in the wake of the doctor who, by this time, is feeling quite cheerful again. Such a situation is by no means uncommon and the important point here is that the chain of events could be broken at any point by any of the participants having enough insight into the true origin of their feelings.

A special case of displacement is represented by the *conversion symptoms* wherein disturbed feelings are displaced into physical channels. Tenseness and inner anxiety, aroused by emotions which we are afraid to recognize, are often displaced into physical symptoms such as headaches, gastric pains, or other bodily discomforts. Many other bodily abnormalities, including constipation, diarrhoea, eruptions of the skin, habitual blushing, and even convulsions, often exist as conversion symptoms in the absence of a purely physical aetiology. Temporary loss of sight, speech, or hearing may even result from a displaced form of emotional disturbance.

Finally, before we leave the mechanism of displacement, it might be worth pointing out that displacement is an established technique of social propaganda. Hitler's persecution of the Jews, for example, gave the German people an opportunity to displace any aggression aroused by the Nazi State on to a substitute object, in this case the Jewish race.

5. Sublimation

Sublimation may be defined as a redirection of repressed impulses into socially acceptable channels. This mechanism is really a further development of displacement, the main distinction being that the sublimated impulses are not merely displaced but redirected into forms of behaviour which are socially useful and acceptable. Sublimation is then a process which aids man in developing his interests and adjusting himself to society. We might say that much of the aggressiveness inherent in human nature is sublimated in competitive games or in the competitive nature of work. Another form of sublimation might be seen in the case of the homosexually inclined individual who successfully sublimates his undesirable feelings into the socially desirable channel of, let us say, being a youth club organizer or a scoutmaster. It has been suggested that nursing provides a source of sublimation for frustrated maternal feelings. Though a useful concept, the idea of sublimation tends to place too much emphasis on the strength and persistence of instincts in influencing all human behaviour. A too general application of this process results in an over-simplification of the complex activities of man. There is little doubt that Charles Lamb's essays or Emily Brontë's novels might have been written somewhat differently had they not remained unmarried. This is merely to say that the shape of a person's life helps to determine the shape of their work. It would be presumptuous to say that, if either of them had been able to find a direct expression of their sexual feelings, then they would not have written anything of note. Some nurses may be unconsciously pouring their thwarted passions into their work but it would seem reasonable to assume that many are merely devoting some of their energies to a useful and interesting job.

6. Rationalization

This process refers to our tendency always to look for a rational explanation to explain our behaviour, although our behaviour may at times be motivated by irrational forces. It has been said, rather aptly, that in rationalizing 'man does not act from reason but reasons from the act'. In other words, we often act on impulses which we prefer to ignore, reassuring ourselves later that we had a logical reason for our action. Probably more than any other personality defence mechanism, rationalization has been taken into every-day speech and the familiar every-day concept of the 'sour grapes' attitude can be seen to be a form of rationalization; the person who fails, let us say, to pass an exam or achieve promotion might rationalize by saying that only 'swots' pass exams and anyway promotion would mean being separated from some of their friends. The social climate of youth would seem to encourage the formation of rationalization. If the child is truthful regarding the reasons for his unacceptable behaviour he is likely to be punished, while if he can give an adequate rationalization he might not only dodge the punishment but also convince himself that he is not such a bad fellow after all. The clinician is again familiar with the abundant rationalizations put forward by patients to account for their symptoms. The amazing facility of the conversion hysteric or hypochondriacal patient in finding organic rationalizations to explain their anxiety feelings is well known. There is little doubt that much of our thinking contains rationalizations which make us able to face many of life's frustrations with self convincing and comforting arguments. Rationalization, particularly if extreme, acts as a barrier to self expression as in the case of people who always find convenient excuses to explain misfortunes which are the result of their own inadequacies.

7. Regression

Regression describes the avoidance of present difficulties by a reversion to an earlier, less mature, way of adjustment to the situation. Some older children, for example, when faced with a difficult situation which makes them anxious, fall back on thumb-sucking behaviour which was the very way in which they relieved inner tension when much younger. The other day a patient described to the writer how her feelings towards her mother had changed greatly since she herself had suffered a nervous breakdown. The patient explained that, where before she enjoyed going out every night with her friends, she now got great comfort out of sitting in the house with her mother at night and how recently she had persuaded her mother to read her stories from a book. This patient clearly described how she had coped with the anxiety aroused by her nervous breakdown by regressing to the way she had behaved as a young child. Extreme cases of regression can be seen in some forms of mental illness, as in the case of a young girl who became so anxious a week before her wedding that she suffered a breakdown during which she acted in every way like a child of 10 years. This regression allowed her for the time to avoid the disturbing situation involved in becoming married. Most adults show regressive behaviour of some degree in stressful situations. The battle-weary and frightened soldier may break down and cry for his mother or even become temporarily enuretic. Illness places the individual under stress of a varying degree and we have already referred to the tendency for patients to regress in their behaviour in hospital by becoming childish and over-dependent in their behaviour. Regression is usually a transient reaction, the individual returning to a more mature way of acting when the stressful situation is alleviated.

Concluding Remarks

An understanding of the nature of unconscious mental activity again argues against the myth that man is a wholly rational animal who is always aware of his actions and the motives which underlie them. At any time we are normally aware of only a portion of the many impulses and feelings which move us to behave in our individual ways. The recognition of unconscious motivation and its implications is not easy to accept, for most of us like to imagine we are always fully in control of our actions. The resistance to accepting that there is more to us than meets even our own eye causes some people to reject completely the importance of unconscious factors. By this denial of what can be conclusively demonstrated the individual only succeeds in limiting his possibilities of insight into his own behaviour and that of others. The opposite reaction is, however, almost equally dangerous. Man may not be the creature of reason we had once imagined, but it would be a mistake to under-value the power of his conscious control over himself and his environment and to picture him as a blind creature whose behaviour is largely dictated by inner forces of which he is unaware. The human race is dominant because it alone has developed the capacity of conscious reasoning which allows man to be creative and to mould his environment actively to his liking. Many of the mechanisms we have discussed involve self-deception but they also have a positive value in aiding us to adjust ourselves to our social environment. We have already argued that a great deal of apparently instinctive behaviour can be easily interpreted as being socially conditioned. We can also take the view that the personality defence mechanisms are products of man's compromise with himself in becoming a member of a civilized society. They are in a sense useful and necessary aids in helping man to live harmoniously with his fellows. If man could achieve complete insight into his own motives and could bring his more primitive unconscious impulses under the control of his conscious reasoning there would be little need for such measures as represion, displacement, projection, and such like. This, however, is an idealistic conception and we must therefore conclude that, by being aware of the existence of unconsciously determined factors in human behaviour, we can at least be a little more able to understand the behaviour of ourselves and others.

QUESTIONS

1. How would you summarize the main differences between conscious and unconscious mental activities? Discuss the influence of unconscious motivation on our everyday behaviour.

2. What is the chief function of the personality defence mechanisms? Comment on any ways in which the mechanisms of rationalization, displacement, and projection might be manifested in the behaviour of both the patient and the nurse.

7. Heredity and Environment

Throughout the previous discussion we have made continual reference to the two basic factors which govern human behaviour. On the one hand we have the indisputable fact that our actions are shaped by social influence, the customs, conventions, and system of values of the society to which we belong. On the other hand we have the equally valid fact that individuals do not passively submit to these influences in a uniform way but react to them in terms of their own unique personality pattern. These two aspects of human motivation can be considered as the influences of environment and heredity respectively. Differences in environment produce an enormous variation of individual differences but some differences exist which appear to be a product of the individual's inheritance rather than of his environment. Contrary to the beliefs expressed in the American Declaration of Independence or in the creed of Soviet Communism, it would seem that all men are not born equal. They are born with different capacities which are in turn acted upon by their environmental experiences to produce the individual personality. The respective influence of inherited and environmental factors exercised the minds of many past students of human behaviour and for some time created an artificial distinction between those who argued that differences in human behaviour were largely governed by differences in inheritance and others who emphasized the importance of environmental differences. This hotly debated issue might be summed up in the question: Is man's destiny decided by the world in which he lives or by what he brings into this world? It will be our purpose in this chapter to demonstrate that neither of these extreme views is valid and that we can never successfully distinguish between the influence of heredity and environment. We shall attempt to demonstrate that the two factors are complementary in their function and than an individual is what he is by virtue of a complex interplay of these two influences.

The Relationship Between Heredity and Environment

If we consider the human being at birth, we can say with a fair degree of certainty that environmental influences are totally absent, unless we include the prenatal and actual birth experiences as environmental. Each of us, then, enters life with a constitution, a genetic pattern, which is made up of inherited factors. As we grow these inherited factors will continue to mature and to influence the course of our development. This basic constitution does not, however, develop in a vacuum but in a world full of stimulation, action, and reaction. Such environmental stimulation is necessary if we are to develop at all as it is the very interplay of constitution and environment which produces the personality of the individual. The inherited endowment of constitution lays down the basic framework of personality and may set down certain limits for its subsequent development. Our environmental experiences, however, continually build up in this framework, deciding the degree to which our inherited capacities will or will not develop, and the particular direction they will take. We might state this briefly by saying that our inherited constitution contains our potentialities while the environment decides to what extent, and in what ways, these potentialities will be realized. Let us follow up this very condensed summary of the complementary relationship between heredity and environment with a more detailed description of how the two factors function in different spheres of personality development.

One aspect of our inherited constitution is that denoted by the term *temperament*. This term is used to designate certain basic personality patterns which are constantly apparent throughout a person's life and are apparently dependent upon the biochemical structure of the individual. Thus certain people exhibit a placid temperament in that they are seldom ruffled or upset even by situations which would disturb others. We might contrast such a person with the volatile person whose emotions are easily aroused and extreme. A person's prevailing mood might be regarded as a feature of temperament in that some people appear to approach every aspect of life with an optimistic and cheerful attitude while others are constantly cautious and pessimistic in their approach. Such general dimensions of personality are closely controlled by body chemistry and the function of the endocrine glands. They can thus be said to be largely hereditary in origin. It would, however, be quite wrong to deduce from this that personality itself is determined by inheritance for we are dealing here only with such simple general factors as the depth and speed of a person's emotional reactions. To explain the unlimited number of ways in which the individual may express his emotional reactions we must take into account all the other environmental influences to which he is exposed. The basic framework of personality may be inherited and innate but it is a plastic framework which may be moulded in a multitude of ways by the different experiences we are subjected to as we develop.

Another suitable illustration of the interplay of heredity and environment is to be found in the sex role which the individual adopts. It would seem a matter of common sense that the question as to whether we will adopt a masculine or feminine role in life will be decided automatically by innate inherited physical-bodily agents such as chromosomes and hormones. Certainly, in the vast majority of cases, the individual accepts the sex role to which he or she is delegated by the physical characteristics at birth. As children we develop certain personality traits which will be either in a masculine or feminine direction according to our physical sex. At puberty the differences between the two sexes become more evident with the maturation of sex organs and the appearance of the secondary sexual characteristics. From this time on the individual will learn to adjust himself or herself to the environment in a predominantly masculine or feminine way and the divergence between the personality traits of the two sexes will widen. Here we might say is a case where the whole development is hereditarily determined and immune to environmental influences. When one studies some of the investigations of this question, however, the answers seem much less conclusive. The anthropologists have shown that many of the personality characteristics we connect with the male or female sex roles are highly susceptible to social influences. Margaret Mead (1935), for example, was given ample evidence to support the view that it is the social, rather than the genetic, pattern which determines the typical male and female modes of behaviour. She studied and described the sex roles in three primitive tribes living within the same one hundred mile area. The first tribe, the Arapesh, are a gentle people with almost complete absence of differentiation in the sex roles. Children of both sexes play together and are brought up in equal measure by both father and mother. Males and females have similar interests, share similar activities, and neither partner is considered the dominant one in the sexual relationship. In the second tribe, the Mundugumor, the pattern is almost completely opposite, both sexes being violent, aggressive, leaving children to fend for themselves. The third tribe, the Tchambuli, show a differentiation in the sex roles which is, however, of a different order than that customarily accepted in our own culture. Here the woman is the active partner both at work and in the sexual relationship. The women work, choose their husband, and are aggressive, boastful, and dominant. The Tchambuli male is submissive, looks after the home and children, and his chief pursuits are in gossiping, wearing bright decorative clothes, and generally endeavouring to make himself attractive to the female. Thus we can see that the assumed biologically determined nature of the sexes is to a great extent socially and culturally derived. Other studies such as that carried out by Terman and Miles (1936) show that even in our own culture the two sexes cannot be clearly differentiated in terms of personality differences. Some men are very feminine in their outlook while some women show many typically masculine habits of behaviour. More recent investigations have suggested that the sex role followed by the individual involves environmental factors which are usually obscured by the fact that, in normal man or woman, the physical sex and the sex role adopted correspond. Three American psychiatrists recently published a paper on a study of the factors which decide the sex role of hermaphrodites (Money *et al.*, 1957). This term refers to people who are born sexually ambiguous, in that their sexual characteristics and physiological make-up are neither exclusively male nor female. Physiological and chemical analysis can show that some of these children are predominantly males with respect to the physical variables of sex, while others are predominantly female. They may at birth, however, appear to be of a neuter gender and the decision taken as to whether they are male or female may often be incorrect. By following up a large series of such cases the authors were able to show that the important factor in deciding the sex role was not the physical sex pattern, but the sex in which the children were reared. Thus one child may grow up to be completely feminine in behaviour and outlook while another child will be psychologically completely masculine, although according to their physical pattern the two children may be female. The authors conclude from their studies that '. . . our findings indicate that neither a purely hereditary nor a purely environmental doctrine of the origins of the gender role and orientation—of physiological sex—is adequate'. Their interpretation of their findings is as follows: 'Rather, it appears that a person's gender role and orientation become established as that person becomes acquainted with and deciphers a continuous multiplicity of signs that point in the direction of his being a boy, or her being a girl. These signs range all the way from nouns and pronouns differentiating gender, to modes of behaviour, hair cut, dress, and personal adornment that are differentiated according to sex' (Money *et al.*, 1957). Thus we must conclude that even such an apparently inherited aspect as the sex role depends a great deal on environmental influences for its development and its direction.

Attempts by psychologists to produce reliable measures of intellectual ability provide another example of the interlinking functions of heredity and environment. One of the most frequent criticisms of standard intelligence tests is that they simply reflect the level of knowledge which the individual has been able to acquire. As this level will obviously depend to a great extent upon the variety of his educational experience, both in the school and in the home, the disadvantaged child will tend to show up badly on such tests. It is clear from a variety of studies that what we call intelligence is not simply a product of education but is also governed by heredity. Should we then speak of two types of intelligence, one a result of education and experience and the other an inherited ability? Some psychologists, such as Hebb (1949), have argued that we cannot speak of two types of intelligence but only of two aspects of intellectual behaviour. He suggests that there are two components in all intellectual behaviour. One is a factor of heredity and is basically the capacity for elaborating perceptions and conceptual activities. The limit of this capacity is constitutionally decided for each individual by the type of brain and nervous system with which he is born. The other component of intelligence consists of permanent changes in the organization of the nerve pathways in the brain and this is a factor of experience. In other words, we can speak of two aspects of intelligence which we might designate as A and B respectively. Each of us is born with certain individual characteristics, such as colour of hair, eyes, body build, etc., which will become more apparent as we develop. This is equally true of intelligence in so far as each of us is born with a brain which by its very structure and organization will set some limit to our intellectual development. Intelligence A thus represents our capacity for development.

Intelligence B on the other hand represents the actual functioning of the brain, the stage of intellectual development actually reached at any age.

The actual stage which any individual does reach will depend not only on his intellectual equipment but also on the extent which he has been able to develop this innate potential. To take a concrete example, we might imagine two children who are born around the same time. The first child may, by virtue of inheritance and other constitutional factors, be born with a brain which is capable of being developed to a very high level. If conditions are right for this child he may be capable of reaching an I.Q. level in adulthood of, let us say, 150. The second child is born with a poorer potential in that his capacity for development is more limited. Let us imagine that the highest level this child could possibly reach in adult life is represented by an I.Q. of 120. Now let us consider what might happen to these two children in their actual development. The first child with a superior potential may be born into a family where education and intellectual stimulation is not encouraged. Let us say that he goes to an over-crowded school, receives little encouragement at home, leaves school at the earliest possible age, and is placed in a job which requires only routine and repetitive work. If we test this person's I.Q. at the age of 25 years, using one of the standard intelligence tests, we may find that his I.Q. is 110. If the second child with the comparatively poorer potential is born into a home where he is encouraged to develop his intellectual resources, is further stimulated at school and goes on to find a job which in itself provides constant intellectual stimulation, we may find in testing him at the age of 25 that his I.Q. is 120. In this case his environment has been such as to allow him to develop his intellectual capacity to its maximum level. We can see from this example, then, that although our intellectual capacity may be to some extent determined for us by factors outside our control, our actual intellectual ability will depend upon the extent to which our environment allows us to make the best of our intellectual equipment. The position for the individual is not, of course, as passive as this description infers. As purposeful human beings we are capable of manipulating and changing our environment to suit our own needs.

For our final illustration of the complementary functions of heredity and environment we turn to consider the response of the human individual to illness. Recent genetic studies have suggested that the tendency to develop tuberculosis is inherited in that some people are constitutionally predisposed towards this illness. This does not, however, throw us back once more to describing tuberculosis as an inherited condition. We now know that such environmental factors as bad housing, malnutrition, and exposure to infection are powerful determinants in the development of tuberculosis. What we may say is that susceptibility of developing a tubercular condition varies according to genetic inheritance, some people having a lower resistance to this illness than others. Whether or not the inherited predisposition results in the person developing the illness will depend entirely upon environmental influences. The same rule may be applied to the major mental illnesses, manic-depressive psychoses and schizophrenia. Studies of both these conditions leave no doubt that they have a genetic component. If, for example, one or two identical twins develops schizophrenia, the likelihood of the other twin becoming schizophrenic is around 65 per cent as compared with the figure of 15 per cent which applies when the twins are not identical and therefore do not have the same hereditary pattern. Some have argued that such findings merely reflect the fact that identical twins are likely to have more shared experiences than non-identical twins. However, studies of identical twins separated at birth and reared in different environments show that the 65 per cent concordance figure for schizophrenia holds up even where the twins have never met.

The artificial distinction between heredity and environment has caused the psychotic group of mental illnesses to be regarded as basically *organic* (constitutional), while the neurotic group of mental illnesses have been regarded traditionally as *functional* (environmental). It is undoubtedly true that the experiences which the individual has to face during his development largely decide whether he will be mentally stable or whether he will display neurotic reactions. War-time studies have shown that, if any individual is faced with prolonged severe and unremitting environmental stress, he will sooner or later suffer some form of mental breakdown (Swank and Marchand, 1946). It is equally true that such reaction to stress is not uniform; some people will break down sooner than others. In fact, people appear to vary a great deal in their capacity to tolerate stress and frustration. Although the factors involved in neurotic breakdown make it impossible to produce statistical evidence, it would seem likely that the capacity to tolerate stress is a constitutional factor, dependent upon inheritance. Studies in the field of the psychoneurosis indicate, for example, that neurotic patients tend to have a lower resistance to physical illness than is normally found in those who do not have a nervous breakdown. Their histories, in fact, suggest that from their earliest days the neurotic patients have shown an exaggerated reaction to any form of physical or mental stress. If this is true then we might again say that the susceptibility to nervous breakdown is an inherited factor, although the appearance or absence of the neurotic reaction will depend upon the type and the severity of the stress which the individual faces in his interaction with his environment.

Concluding Remarks

The effects of heredity and environment on our development are virtually indistinguishable. Inheritance sets some limit on each individual's development but it leaves a very broad range of possibilities open. The extent to which these possibilities are realized will depend largely upon the environmental influences to which we are exposed. Although we then depend a great deal on the type of environment in which we develop we cannot conclude that we are passively moulded by environmental influences beyond our control. Each individual rather interacts with his environment, changing it and actively organizing it to suit his own purposes. What we are today is not dependent upon our inherited constitution or our social environment, but rather upon the way in which we have manipulated our environment to make the best possible use of our individual capacities.

QUESTIONS

1. Discuss the difficulties of making a clear cut distinction between the contribution of heredity on one hand and environment on the other to personality development.

2. Comment on the influence of inherited and environmental factors on the development of intelligence. To what extent is the I.Q. the product of a person's education, relative to his inherited intellectual capacity?

8. Environmental Stimulation

From infancy onwards throughout life we are constantly exposed to an ever-changing array of stimuli from our environment. Such environmental stimulation, as we have seen, is vital in allowing us to develop our latent capacities. Much attention has already been directed to the deleterious effects of over-stimulation where the individual collapses under the stress of the complexities of modern living. Any machine has an optimal working capacity and if it is pushed adequate performance. Although it is dangerous to push the analogy between man and machine too far, it is equally true that human beings react in adverse ways if they are forced to make too many decisions at once, or in any way to perform beyond their capabilities. Like the machine, people may suffer a breakdown if exposed to an over-demanding environment for a sustained period without at least a temporary respite. Each summer we enjoy the beneficial effects of a holiday after the accumulated stress and strain of the past year. The essential feature of a holiday is that it provides not only a rest, but a change from the normal day-to-day routine. Recently we have become more aware of the human organisms' need for change and our susceptibility to monotony and lack of stimulation. Although it is true to say that individuals may become disturbed because their environment is too stimulating and demanding, it appears to be equally true that we may become disturbed because our environment is monotonous and lacking in stimulation. Indeed, our everyday experience contains many illustrations of people actively seeking stressful forms of stimulation from their environment. Such sources of stimulation vary widely, from the harmless thrill of the 'Big Wheel' at the fairground, to climbing unconquered mountains or watching horror films.

Psychiatrists who are concerned with the treatment of the milder forms of neurotic reactions have noticed that some of their patients complain, not of too much stress in their life, but of too little. Their symptoms appear to develop in a context of boredom and monotony. As a current example of this, we might refer to the term 'suburban neurosis' which has been used to refer to a common neurotic syndrome typical of young, usually middle-class mothers, who have settled in the suburbs with a young family to rear. The symptoms shown by this group include complaints of irritability, lack of appetite, generalized anxiety and mild depression. These symptoms, although distressing to the individual, are temporary and usually disappear very quickly after the youngest child starts school. Such patients are usually young, intelligent and well-educated women who have been working in an interesting and stimulating job before marriage. After marriage they move into a new area where they have yet to make friends and the arrival of infants on the scene further restricts their activities. Much of the day is spent within the four walls of a home, with young children as their only human contact. It would seem that their symptoms arise as a result of being temporarily deprived of the sources of stimulation to which they have been accustomed.

Living and working in the hubbub of modern civilization, most people probably find their environment stimulating enough. We are constantly bombarded by a bewildering variety of noise, colour, and other sensory experiences; continually asked to make decisions. We may feel that it would be a welcome relief to find ourselves in a situation in which our brains were asked to do a great deal less. In the remainder of this chapter we will consider some investigations into the reactions of people when placed in artificial experimental conditions in which normal environmental stimulation is greatly reduced. We shall also consider a more naturally occurring phenomenon which also involves a reduction in sensory intake—the state of sleep.

Performance Under Monotonous Conditions

The subject of fatigue and its effect have for long been of interest to psychologists, particularly those who have applied themselves to industrial problems. From such studies we have accumulated a great deal of knowledge regarding the detrimental effects of fatigue on human performance. The main effects of fatigue are lack of concentration, slowness in thinking, mood changes such as irritability, and temporary changes in the level of consciousness. Very similar effects can sometimes occur when the individual is not physically tired but is faced with a situation which is monotonous and lacking in change.

Although automation and other technical developments in industry have resulted in machines carrying out many of the routine and monotonous tasks which once required a human operator, there are many types of work which still involve monotonous conditions. In some jobs the operator's main task is to monitor the performance of automated machines, keeping a sustained vigil over the movements of dials and gauges which express the machine's performance. Many of the experimental studies of monotonous conditions have reproduced such conditions by presenting subjects with tasks which demand the constant monitoring of signals over a substantial period of time. Thus the subject might be required to watch a pointer moving slowly around a clock face. From time to time the pointer makes a movement which is twice as long as the standard movement, and the subject's task is to press a lever when this is observed. In this, and in many similar types of experiments, it has been shown that a decline in the accuracy of the subject's performance is evident within the first half hour of the task. As the time goes on, more errors tend to be made, these consisting mainly of the subject missing the signal to which he was meant to respond. If the intervals between the appropriate signals are fairly regular, the subject may take advantage of this fact by spacing his lapses of attention so that they occur when the signal is unlikely to appear. The decline in performance may also be lessened by introducing into the situation any new feature which will ease the monotony. Apart from the objective evidence of poorer performance observed by subjects in such conditions, the subjective reports of the subjects themselves indicate that a monotonous repetitive task such as this induces feelings of irritability, restlessness, boredom, and day-dreaming. Indeed, the monotonous nature of such tasks may quickly produce such a state of fatigue as to cause momentary lapses of consciousness akin to sleep. Some such studies have used the EEG, or to give its fully impressive and unpronounceable title, the electroencephalogram. The EEG picks up, amplifies and records the electrochemical discharges from the brain which are found to vary in pattern according to the level of consciousness of the subject. Thus, while one pattern of rhythm is characteristic of the alert waking state, another is characteristic of the sleeping state, while other patterns correspond to intermediary levels of consciousness. Oswald (1960) has shown that the effects of rhythmical and monotonous stimulation (slowly flashing lights and soft music) eventually induced sleep in his subjects—even when they had their eyes taped back so that they could not be closed. Long before sleep is actually induced, however, the subjects show momentary lapses of consciousness of periods of a second or two. A significant fact about such transient changes in consciousness is that the subject is himself unaware of them, imagining himself to be alert throughout. One can see that in any job where constant vigilance is imperative, the effects of monotony could be in fact more dangerous than that of complete fatigue. If we are extremely tired and exhausted, we are aware of our condition and will probably take this into consideration before attempting tasks which demand a high level of attention and accuracy. The effects of monotony on performance are less subjectively noticeable and therefore the probability of dangerous error is greater. In nursing, for example, we might think of night duty when the normal changing stream of sensory stimuli are greatly reduced and the nurse has to stay alert in an atmosphere of muted light and sound. One might visualize situations here where even a momentary lapse of alertness might lead to serious consequences.

A notable example of such a situation occurs in the intensive care units where the nurse's task may be to monitor physiological recorders (e.g. ECG's) for signs of abnormal function. The strain of continual vigilance in conditions during the night is almost certain to lead to important signals being missed.

Sensory Deprivation

Although most of us may have experienced monotonous conditions such as those described above, it is seldom that the normal flow of sensory stimulation from the environment falls below a certain minimum level. In the last few years there have been some interesting studies of the reactions of human beings to experimental environments which are carefully controlled to reduce sensory stimulation well below the normal level.

There are numerous reports of the unusual and unpleasant experiences of normal individuals exposed to unusual environmental conditions. Full and interesting accounts have been written by explorers, shipwrecked mariners and others who have recalled their traumatic experiences in detail. Although the experiences of such people differ, most of them report that the most frightening aspect of their ordeal was the dreadful *sameness* of the environment and the persistent monotony of being exposed to an unchanging pattern of stimuli for a length of time. People have been known to break down on polar expeditions, not through the physical hardships involved, but through the effects of being isolated from all the normal visual and auditory stimulation missing in the white silent polar spaces. Admiral Byrd expresses this feeling in the following extract from his reports: 'I feel a tremendous need for stimuli from the outside world and yearn for sounds, smells, voices, and touch. . . . I want terribly to have someone who could confirm any impression or, better still, argue about them. I began to feel that I would be incapable of discerning between the false and the true' (quoted from Wexler *et al.*, 1957). The common element in most of the situations reported is that the environmental conditions involve a reduction in the normal pattern of stimuli, sights, and sounds, which are so commonplace as to make us unaware of their importance. In recent years some psychologists have devised experimental conditions of 'sensory deprivation' where volunteers are exposed to an environment in which normal environmental stimulation is reduced to a minimal degree. Hebb (1955) and his colleagues at McGill University in Canada studied volunteer students who were isolated in a specially designed air-conditioned room. The subjects wore a special form of suiting, complete with ear-plugs and translucent goggles, which cut off their normal sensory contact with the environment. Exposure to such an artificial environment for a length of time resulted in a decided change in the subjects' experiences. Their thinking became confused, their concentration impaired, and, in some cases, vivid hallucinations were experienced. A later worker in America (Lilly, 1956) made this type of experiment more disturbing by immersing the subjects in a tank containing slowly flowing water at body temperature. This experiment was arranged in such a way that the subjects could not see, hear, or have any sense of pressure, movement, or touch. The effect of being suspended in water also greatly reduced the normal body-pressure imposed by gravity. It is difficult to imagine a more monotonous environment than this situation in which practically all sensory stimulation is absent. The results were similar to those found in Hebb's experiment, although more exaggerated and more disturbing for the subjects involved. Another report of sensory deprivation (Mendelson and Foley, 1956) comes from an observation made on a group of patients being treated for poliomyelitis in a new tank-type of respirator. In this respirator vision is greatly restricted, the patient lying constantly in the same position and hearing nothing apart from the rhythmic sounds of the respirator motor and bellows. This apparatus, designed as an improvement on the usual type of respirator used in polio treatment, had to be considerably modified simply because the patients could not be induced to stay in the respirator for longer than twenty-four hours. They again found the situation terrifying and reported similar effects to that found in other experiments involving deliberately induced sensory deprivation.

From this type of work we might conclude that our very hold on reality is basically dependent upon us receiving a continual and uninterrupted flow of sensory stimulation from our environment. Hebb's own remarks regarding these investigations imply the same conclusion: 'The well-adjusted adult therefore is not intrinsically less subject to emotional disturbance: he is well adjusted, relatively unemotional, as long as he is in his cocoon (his cultural environment). We think of some persons as being emotionally dependent and others not; but it looks as though we are completely dependent upon the environment in a way and to a degree that we have not suspected' (Hebb, 1955).

It needs little imagination to apply these findings to the hospital patient whose illness may place him in a situation which involves a severe restriction of the normal pattern of sensory stimulation. Consider, for example, a patient suffering from an eye injury, lying for a length of time in an isolated room with his normal visual contact with the environment reduced by protective bandages. Patients deprived in this way often give the impression of being 'hungry' for stimuli, welcoming any sound or any activity which keeps them in touch with the outside world. It is also worth noting that many of the reactions occurring in these sensory deprivation experiments appear to be due as much to the enforced immobility of the subject as to the reduction in external stimulation. It seems likely that normally physical movement provides the nervous system with a certain level of stimulation which may compensate for any reduction in the normal flow of stimulation from the outside world. It is certainly true that people often react to monotony with restlessness and obtain some relief by physical movement.

Such detrimental effects of immobility should perhaps be kept in mind when we consider the case of the hospital patient who is forced by his illness to lie in bed for considerable periods of time. It would appear that bed-sores are only one of the harmful effects of the enforced immobility experienced by the chronically ill patient.

Exposure to a non-stimulating environment is not the only stress faced by subjects in sensory deprivation experiments. The passive nature of the situation denies subjects the normal repertoire of responses which normally aid us in coping with our environment. However, in some situations the individual may cease to respond adequately to his environment simply because he has learned that his responses are of little or no consequence. Such a psychological state, where one perceives oneself to have no control over one's destiny, has been termed 'learned helplessness'.

This concept evolved from animal studies of the effects of exposure to aversive stimuli upon subsequent behaviour. Seligman (1975) observed that dogs continually placed in experimental conditions where they were unable to escape noxious stimuli like electric shocks developed a curiously passive behavioural pattern. When subsequently placed in a situation allowing easy escape from shocks, they did not initiate any of the usual avoidance behaviours; instead, they submitted themselves passively to the traumatic stimuli. In addition, the general passive sluggish and apathetic demeanour of these experimental animals suggested a state similar to depression. Generalizing his findings, Seligman theorised that any organism subjected to repeated exposure to situations in which its responses have no effect upon the outcome of the forces impinging upon it actually develops a state of learned helplessness, which is similar to a reactive depression. Subsequent works with human subjects (e.g. Glass and Singer, 1972) has tended to support this view in demonstrating similar stress reactions in humans exposed to noxious stimulation over which they have no control. It has been demonstrated that, in such situations, both psychological and physiological components of stress reactions may be greatly reduced if the subject is given the opportunity of perceiving himself to have some control over the situation. Thus, in one study, subjects were able to withstand more severe electric shocks and show fewer stress reactions to them if they were given a 'panic button' which, when pressed, would lessen the intensity of the shocks. An important aspect here is that the control need only be perceived rather than actual. Subjects in this study showed a reduction in stress reactions when the panic button was available, even though they did not utilize it during the experiment. Since these studies were reported, a number of investigations have claimed the successful alleviation of depressive symptoms by teaching people various strategies aimed at increasing their perception of having more control over their life situations.

It certainly seems likely that the complexities of today's society may cause many of its members to feel that they are passive, helpless pawns whose own convictions and behaviours cannot alter the events surrounding them. We have already suggested that illness and hospitalization may be potent factors in incurring feelings of passivity and helplessness. Another environmental situation which, in the author's experience, is likely to engender a maximum degree of learned helplessness is incarceration in a large institution such as a penitentiary. Here, regardless of how humane the system, the individual is invariably led to perceive himself as a non-person, a number, whose responses have very little influence on his day-to-day environment.

If we wish to avoid a heightened level of depressive reactions in such situations, it would seem imperative that every possible opportunity be taken to increase the individual's sense of personal control and thereby to reduce the debilitating effects of perceiving one's self as a passive, helpless component of a powerful system.

Sleeping

We have already discussed some of the reactions of human subjects to experimentally controlled conditions where the level of environmental stimulation is greatly reduced. There is, however, a naturally occurring state of reduced stimulation to which all of us are subject—the state of sleep. It is perhaps surprising to realize that, if we live to the age of 75, we will have spent somewhere around 25 years of our life sleeping. Most healthy people tend to take for granted that each morning they will wake refreshed after their normal quota of around eight hours' restful slumber. If, because of the nature of our work, domestic disturbances or any personal reason, our normal sleep rhythm is temporarily disturbed we quickly find that not only is our general efficiency lowered, but that we feel lethargic, irritable and sadly lacking in our normal zest and enthusiasm. Many unfortunate people find that habitual insomnia can be an extremely difficult problem and our dependence on a good night's sleep has made fortunes for the manufacturers of sleep-inducing drinks and pills. But what is a good night's sleep? Although we tend to take the magical eight hours as being the answer here, a short survey of the sleep habits of our friends may quickly suggest that some people get by very well on considerably less than eight hours, while others appear to require more. We may notice that as people get older they will say that they do not need as much sleep as before. Perhaps we could begin this brief survey of sleep by considering how the sleep rhythm does change with age.

Changes in the Sleep Pattern with Age

If we wanted to obtain some idea as to whether, and in what direction, sleep habits change with age, we might conduct a little private experiment by asking a number of friends of different ages about their sleep. Such a privately conducted survey might provide us with a tentative answer to our question, but most of us would unfortunately find our circle of friends too limited to afford us a large enough sample to make such a survey worth while. Some psychologists have carried out similar surveys on larger samples of people specially selected so that their responses give us a clearer idea of the sleep habits of the population as a whole. If we take large enough samples of different age groups and simply ask them how long they usually sleep, we receive answers which are illustrated in Figure 3.

Figure 3

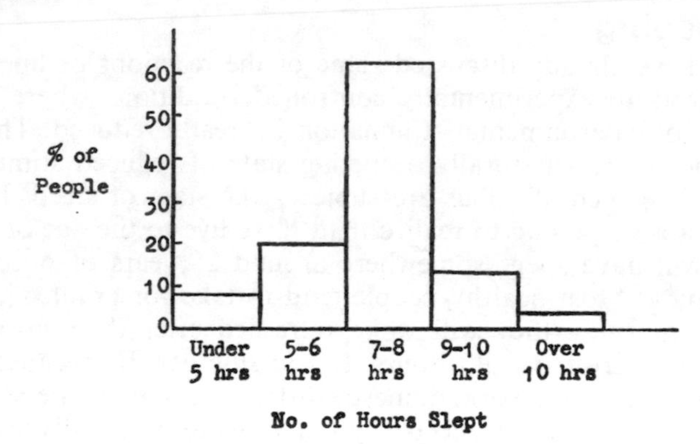

In this particular survey (McGhie and Russell, 1962) it can be seen that the majority (62 per cent) of people said that they normally slept between seven and eight hours. However, quite a number of people (about 23 per cent in this survey) said that they sleep considerably less than this, while a very fortunate one person in every 50 boasted of an average evening's sleep of over 10 hours. If we break down our sample into different age groups, it quickly becomes obvious that most people sleep less as they grow older. To illustrate this we might refer to Figure 4 which represents the percentage of people at each age group complaining of insomnia.

Figure 4

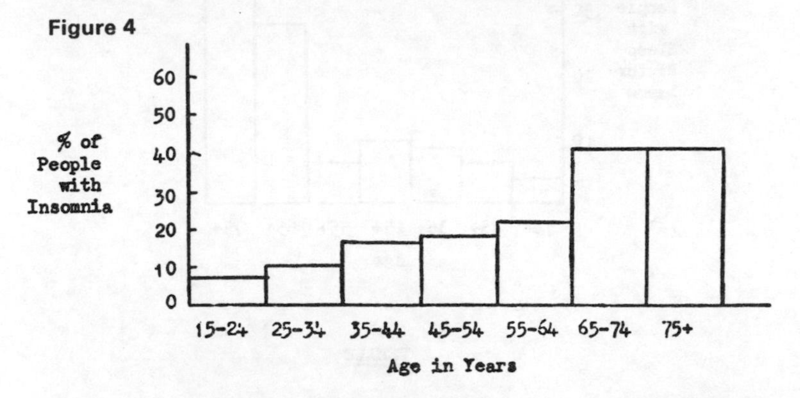

It can be seen from this diagram that insomnia is reported with increasing frequency as age advances. It is worth noting here that, although more older people describe sleep difficulties, complaints of being tired in the morning are more often reported by young people. This may mean that as we grow older we sleep less, simply because we need less sleep.

Surprisingly enough, some such surveys of sleep habits suggest differences in sleep not only among different age groups but between the two sexes. Insomnia is reported much more frequently by women than by men up to the age of about 65 years. The difference between the male and the female sleep pattern is most easily illustrated in Figure 5 (overleaf).

It can be seen from Figure 5 that the frequency of insomnia in males is comparatively low until the age of 65 years when there is a sudden increase. Sleep difficulties in the female increase more consistently with age and are well established by middle age. As the age of 65 years is the normal retiral age for men, the sudden disturbance in the sleep rhythm at this time may reflect the disruption of normal daily habits consequent to stopping work.

Sleep and Temperament

Why is it that at times we find we get off to sleep without any trouble, while at other times we toss and turn for what seems an eternity before falling asleep? There can of course be fairly obvious physical reasons for a disturbed night's

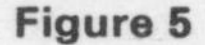
Figure 5

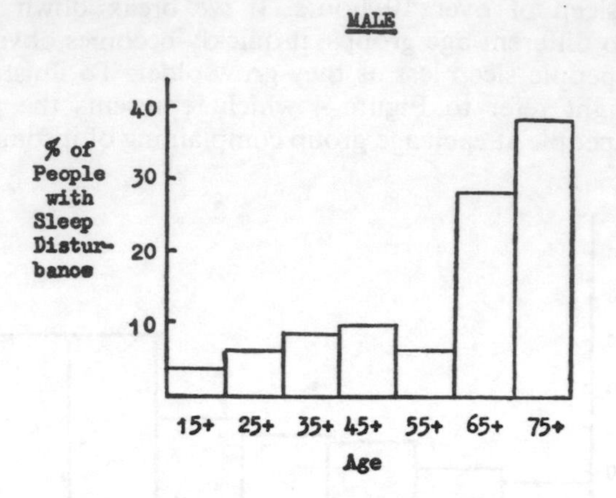

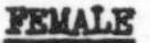

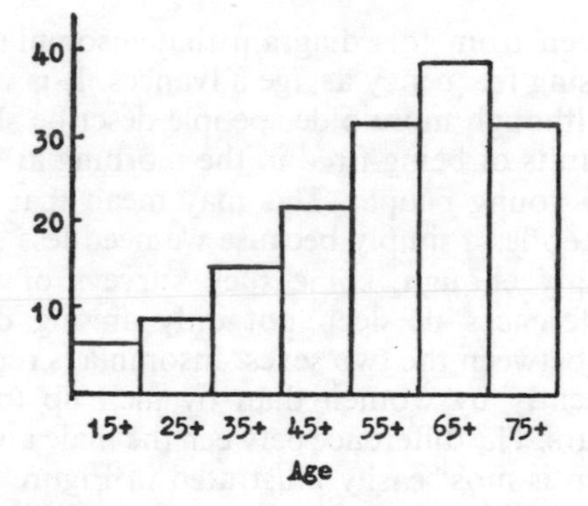

sleep, particularly when this follows an enjoyable but unwisely heavy supper. It is also true, however, that our sleep rhythm is particularly sensitive to our current emotional and mental state. Indeed, severe disturbance of the sleep rhythm is a very common complaint of people under treatment for a nervous breakdown. Most of us have probably already recognized that anxiety and worry may cause insomnia. If we are unfortunate enough to be of a worrying nature, our chronically tense and anxious attitude may cause us to join the ranks of the habitual insomniac. The sleeping pills which are sought by an increasingly higher percentage of modern society usually act by reducing our anxiety and thus allowing natural sleep to follow.

Some psychologists have attempted to link differences in sleep habits with other aspects of the individual temperament. Perhaps one of the most distinct ways in which people differ in this respect is not in the manner in which they sleep, but rather the manner in which they awaken. Some people always appear to waken up very quickly in the morning, feeling alert and bright and eager to face a new day. Others (the present author among them) struggle awake only after an intense conflict, and spend the first hour of each morning in a state of mental and physical incoordination and lethargy. One might imagine with horror the friction that must result when two such extreme types marry. I remember a female patient telling me how her feelings towards her husband had changed irrevocably on the first morning of her honeymoon, when she discovered it was his habit to spring from bed singing, and spend the next 15 minutes happily exercising in front of an open window. There is some suggestion that such different reactions to sleep and wakening may be partially dependent upon the bodily chemistry and constitution of the individual. It has been suggested, for example, that such temperamental differences are related to the bodily build of the individual and that people with a thin, long physique are more likely to be at their best in the evening and at their lowest ebb first thing in the morning. In contrast to this, people with a heavier, more rotund body build are more likely to be among the ranks of those who are likely to shatter their sleeping partner's nerves with a rousing chorus of 'Oh what a beautiful morning'. Perhaps all engaged couples should be encouraged to sleep together at least once before marriage, to establish that they are good at getting *out* of bed together.

Dreaming

Back in the Dark Ages, when the present author was a boy, there was a popular song entitled, 'I'm a dreamer, aren't we all?' Many people would reply in the negative to the implication here, asserting that they seldom, if ever, dream. They might justifiably react with incredulity if told that we all enjoy roughly the same ration of dreams each and every night. Yet this is but one of a series of assertions which have now been made by physiologists and psychologists who have recently invaded the private territory of our dream-life. In our earlier discussion of unconscious motivation, we referred to Freud's interest in the dream as an expression of activity in the unconscious part of the mind. Indeed, since Freud first published his interpretation of dreams in 1900, the process of dreaming has been of great interest to psychologists. In describing the dream as 'the royal road into the unconscious,' Freud argued that the dream was composed of wishes and longings of which the individual was normally not conscious in his waking life. During sleep, the guard or 'censorship' which normally separates the conscious and the unconscious sectors of the mind is lowered to allow unconscious impulses to slip through in the form of dreams. As Freudian theory regarded the unconscious as being composed mainly of sexual or aggressive drives, the dream was thus seen to be a sort of safety valve which allowed the individual to express his antisocial wishes, if only in a phantasy form. Many of us, reflecting on the unexciting and relatively respectable nature of our own dreams, may wonder if Freud was unusually fortunate in his dream repertoire. In this theory of dreams it was maintained however that the events we recall in our dreams are only symbols which have to be interpreted before the real meaning of the dream becomes evident. It was also argued that we hide from ourselves the true meaning behind our dreams by conveniently forgetting or 'repressing' a great deal of the content of our dreams. Thus the difference between the frequent and the infrequent dreamer would seem to be one of accessibility of recall. According to this argument then, the less we remember dreaming, the less respectable and self-acceptable can our dreams have been.

Although the process of dreaming has retained its interest for psychologists, it was not until very recently that any significant advance was made in our understanding of the dream process. The main difficulty in studying dreams lies of course in the private and subjective nature of the process of dreaming itself. The recent widening in our understanding of dreams has come about chiefly through technical advances which have provided us with more reliable and objective indices of dreaming. These studies began with an accidental observation that from time to time while asleep, the eyes move rapidly from left to right in a series of brief scanning movements. By means of a device which monitors these rapid eye movements (REM's) and records their appearance and duration on the EEG, it was possible to assess their distribution and to question their significance. The sporadic presence of the rapid eye movements (REM's) together with associated changes in the brain's activity as recorded on the EEG, suggested the possibility that these represented dream activity. Further investigations showed that, when people are wakened immediately after rapid eye movements occur, they declare that they have been wakened during a dream. When, on the other hand, they are wakened when no rapid eye movements have occurred, they deny having been dreaming. Such findings give sufficient support for the conclusion that the act of dreaming is accompanied by rapid movements of the eyes, as if the dreamer were actually visually scanning his own dream. Once such a reasonably reliable measure of the presence of dreams is available, we can begin to test out some of the past theories regarding dreams.

If, for example, we use the EEG to tell us the depth at which the individual is sleeping at any moment, and at the same time measure the appearance of dreams as indicated by rapid eye movements, we find that dreams tend to occur at the lighter levels of sleep. Figure 6 illustrates the way in which dreams are associated with the sleep rhythm.

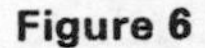

Figure 6

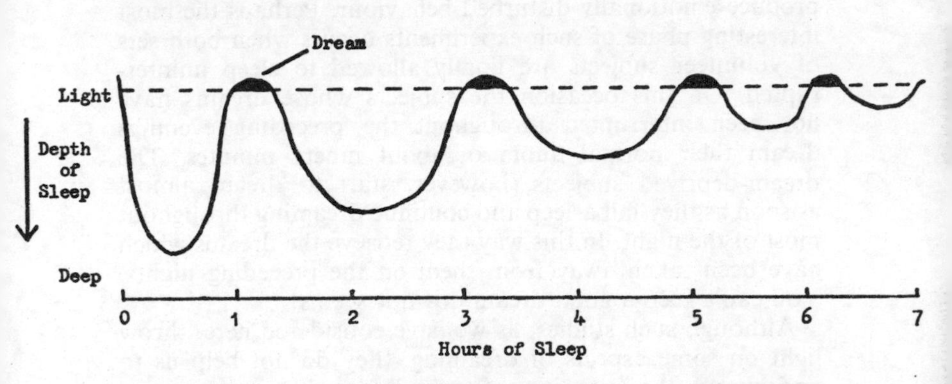

The findings of those scientists who have investigated dream activity strongly suggest that, not only do we all dream every night, but that the proportion of sleeping time spent in dreams varies little from person to person. On the average we seem to spend about 80 to 90 minutes per night in dreaming, this period being broken up into a number of separate dreams. It will be remembered that Freud had earlier suggested that dreaming was a therapeutic process which allowed us to discharge our frustrations harmlessly in sleep. Taking this view we might expect that, if anything were to happen to deny us this outlet, our mental state would suffer. Now that it is possible to chart objectively the occurrence of dreams, we can conduct the rather bizarre experiment of depriving people of their dreams and noting their reactions. The experiment here simply consists of taking two groups of volunteers and depriving one group of their normal night's quota of dreams by wakening them for a few seconds immediately rapid eye movements have been observed, thus effectively interrupting the dream. The remaining subjects are wakened also for an equivalent number of very brief periods throughout the night, but never when rapid eye movements are observed. In other words, their dreaming time is not affected. If we keep this process going for about four or five nights, we find that the dream-deprived subjects report changes in their behaviour which are also clearly apparent to others. They feel irritable, apprehensive, anxious, mildly depressed, and describe themselves as 'on edge'. The non-dream-deprived subjects on the other hand report no change in their personality and there is no observable indication of any alteration in their behaviour. Thus it can be said that being deprived of the normal ration of dreams for a few nights is enough to produce emotionally disturbed behaviour. Perhaps the most interesting phase of such experiments occurs when both sets of volunteer subjects are finally allowed to sleep uninterrupted. On this occasion the subjects whose dreams have not been interrupted throughout the preceding evenings dream their normal quota of about ninety minutes. The dream-deprived subjects, however, start to dream almost as soon as they fall asleep and continue dreaming throughout most of the night. In this way they retrieve the dreams which have been taken away from them on the preceding nights. You can't keep a good dream down it seems!

Although such studies, as we have considered here, throw light on some aspects of dreaming, they do not help us to understand the meaning of our dreams. Dreams are in essence pictorial representations of our own thoughts. Introspective studies such as that reported by Silberer (1912) demonstrate that, as we become more tired, our thoughts tend to take more of a visual form—being experienced as images or pictures in our mind. In a state of relaxed fatigue, we also find that our 'picture thoughts' arise in our mind and run their course largely outside of our conscious control. They seem to have a life of their own. Another characteristic of thinking when we are tired is the symbolic nature of our thoughts. Ideas and words are represented by visual images which are somewhat indirect and distorted in their meaning. Thus, if we are dwelling on our current difficulties we might find this being represented by an image of ourselves trying to climb out of a deep hole. As dreams are associated with relatively light levels of sleep, they can probably be regarded as more vivid examples of the type of visual thinking which occurs in the relaxed fatigued state. Another factor here is that, when tired or asleep, we are shutting out the normal flow of sensory stimulation from the outside world, thus causing ourselves to dwell more on internal and personal thoughts.

However, as we have already suggested, our contact with the external world is never completely cut off, even in sleep. The content of some of our dreams may reflect changes in our immediate environment while we sleep. A radical change in the temperature of our surroundings may cause us to dream—let us say of Arctic exploration. Noises, such as the ringing of an alarm clock, may be incorporated into a dream, so removing the necessity of wakening. Some careful studies (*e.g.* Berger, 1963) have been made of the extent to which the content of dreams may be altered by verbal stimuli repeatedly played over to the sleeping subject. These investigations show that the sleeping subject may incorporate such verbal stimuli into his dream, but in a slightly modified way. Thus repetition of the name 'Gillian' caused one subject to dream of an old woman from Chile (a Chilean). Another subject dreamed of a distorted rabbit, after the name 'Robert' was repeatedly presented during sleep.

Concluding Remarks

Here we have considered some of the ways in which we react to changes in the relationship between ourselves and the outside world. We might regard our brain as an infinitely complex mechanism for dealing with information reaching us from the external environment. It is continually processing the continual stream of information relayed by our sense organs. If we ask it to operate beyond its maximal capacity, its performance may be less accurate. When circumstances are such that the brain and nervous system are starved of the normal level of environmental stimulation, a similar falling off in the brain's efficiency occurs. Such reduction in sensory contact with the outside world causes our thinking to be less rational, less orientated to reality, reflecting more our inner drives and strivings which are normally controlled and outside of conscious awareness. Such changes may occur when we are overtired, bored, isolated from the outside world, or when we are asleep.

QUESTIONS

1. Discuss the effects on human behaviour of a monotonous and restricted environment.

2. To what extent do modern studies of sleep and dreaming clarify our understanding of these processes?

Part Three
Interaction with the Environment

Thus far we have discussed the development of the human personality and the various types of factors which motivate human behaviour. In this and the following chapters we will be concerned with the ways in which we become aware of our environment and interact with it. In other words, we will now be directly concerned with examining the processes which govern human behaviour. These include the processes of attending, perceiving, learning, remembering, and thinking. Each of these processes has been the subject of a great deal of psychological investigation and our consideration of them will of necessity be brief and incomplete. The general theme throughout the succeeding chapters will be that such mental processes do not function passively according to set rules, but involve and are influenced by the whole personality of the individual who adjusts himself to his environment in an active way.

9. The Processes of Attending and Perceiving

Attending

Before we can interact with our environment we must first be aware of it. Through our various senses we receive stimuli from the environment which allow us to become aware of the world outside ourselves and to behave in certain ways in relation to it. At any one time there are an immense number of stimuli in the outside world which impinge upon our senses. We do not, of course, take all these stimuli in at once, but rather select certain stimuli and ignore others. This process of selection is, of course, what we normally mean when we speak of attention. When we attend to anything in our environment we narrow the range of our awareness so as to focus it upon some specific item. As we have already indicated, however, attention also has marginal aspects in that, although we may be concentrating out attention on one specific event, we are often more dimly aware of other events which lie, as it were, on the margin of our attention. Very often we remember things later which at the time we did not seem to be attending to, thus demonstrating that even events which occur outside the direct field of our attention may be taken in and influence our behaviour. We have already described attention as an active process but it is also a constant process. Although the teacher may criticize his pupils for not 'attending' we can be certain that the class is attending to something, although it may not be their lesson. We are never in a position of existing in a vacuum. Even if we withdraw all our attention from our environment we will still be attending to our inner thoughts. The question then arises as to what principles guide our selection of certain factors in our environment to the exclusion of others.

Knowledge of the principles involved here is of great

practical value in such fields as advertising but we need not describe these in great detail here. Certain stimuli in the environment are more attention-demanding in that they have qualities which attract our attention. Such qualities include the strength of the stimulus, repetition of the stimulus, change, novelty, and incongruity. Thus, for example, a loud noise will attract attention more easily than a soft one, as will a noise which is repeated until it forces us to attend. The quality of change is well illustrated in the neon light type of advertising and many advertisements also use the attention-demanding value of novelty in presentation. However, the most important factors which influence our attention are not qualities of the stimuli themselves but qualities of the individual personality. Other things being equal, we will attend to anything which fits in with our current interests and basic needs. Again such facts are well known to advertisers who seek to present their advertisements in a form which will appeal to the needs and interests of potential customers. The fact that the sexually stimulating advertisement is one of the most commonly used is perhaps a sad reflection upon the needs of modern man.

Attention, then, is an active selective process whereby the individual chooses from the mass of competing stimuli in his environment the particular stimuli which fit in with his personal needs. One practical lesson we might draw from this is that attention will be easier and more concentrated the less competition there is from other competing stimuli.

The student who maintains that he studies better when surrounded by such distractions as a blaring radio, others talking, and so forth, is usually rationalizing. There are some conditions in which distraction may be beneficial. We have already discussed the deleterious effects of monotony upon attention and performance in general. If we are required to sustain our attention on a task which is intrinsically boring, some degree of external stimulation may help to keep us sufficiently alert. On occasions when we are over-anxious or preoccupied with personal worries, our attempt to concentrate our attention on external tasks may be distracted by our disturbed inner mental state. Indeed, one of the most common complaints of people suffering from nervous disorder is of an inability to concentrate. In some of the more severe forms of mental illness this loss of control over their attention is very marked. The deeply depressed patient cannot attend to everyday events in the outside world because his attention is fully occupied with his inner melancholia, thoughts, and feelings. The term 'melancholia,' which was once used by psychiatrists to denote severe depression, means literally 'full-up,' and aptly describes a state of inner morbid preoccupation in which the outside world is effectively shut out. Although (at one time) it was thought the schizophrenic patient's withdrawn state signified a similar turning away of attention from the world, more recent studies suggest that the disorder of attention shown by these patients takes the opposite form—at least in the early stages of their illness. Such studies (Payne and Hewlett, 1960; McGhie and Chapman, 1961, 1962; McGhie, 1965) demonstrate that the young schizophrenic patient experiences an inability to attend selectively to the many outside stimuli which compete for his attention. His general performance suffers because he cannot exclude anything going on in his environment, whether it is relevant or irrelevant to the task in hand. At this stage of his illness the schizophrenic patient does not ignore his environment although he is continually distracted by it. It is possible that the completely withdrawn and uncommunicative state of such patients in the more chronic stage of a schizophrenic illness represents their only defence against an environment which is overwhelming in its impact.

Perceiving

After we have attended to anything we 'take it in' and give it a meaning. This process of assimilating stimuli in a meaningful and organized way is known as 'perceiving', Once again the important principle governing perception is that we do not passively perceive like a camera but rather actively organize our perceptions in our own individual way. The meaning and significance we give to anything perceived is dependent not only upon the object itself but upon our past experiences and our future expectations; *e.g.*, if a wife points out a red stain on her husband's jacket he may perceive this as being blood if he had cut himself while shaving that morning, or as lipstick if his morning's activities had taken a different form. The young mother relaxing in the evening may perceive any strange noise as being her baby crying upstairs. Her perception of the stimuli will be influenced by her current state of mind. In fact, the way we perceive things depends a great deal upon our individual personality. A class of students may receive the same lecture but the meaning they take out of it will depend upon their individual attitudes and outlook.

As perceptions of external stimuli are so greatly influenced by individual personal factors it follows that there is every chance that different people may perceive the same object or situation in different ways. It is a well-known fact, for example, that the testimony of different witnesses to the same event varies so greatly as to be almost valueless. For example, a number of people witnessing a car accident may vary greatly in their reports as to the events leading up to the accident. To take one aspect of this, some of the male witnesses may see the accident as having been the fault of the female driver and some of the witnesses present, who are themselves drivers of cars, may see it as the fault of the pedestrian. It might be quite true, then, to say that no two people attending to the same object actually perceive it in an identical way. Once again we must conclude that if we wish to act efficiently as an observer of the behaviour of other people and to make judgments about people in general, we must be as fully aware as possible of the influence of aspects of our own personality upon what we observe. We might also conclude that no two people ever can be said to share the same experience because they perceive the experience differently. We can thus never explain a person's present actions fully, merely on the basis of what has happened to him in the past, without also considering the meaning which the individual has given to his past experiences. Returning to our example of a class of students listening to a lecture, we might say that the lecture will be of great value to some of the class because these students have been able to invest the content of the lecture with a meaning and significance in terms of their own personal experience. Other students who have not been able to do this will perceive less value in the material that they have been given. We will return to this fact when we discuss the process of learning but we might note here that it is of importance that the lecturer should take pains to relate his material to the personal experiences of his class and ensure that, as far as possible, each of them has perceived what he has said in the same way. As we have already stated, the dependence of perception upon personal factors means that perceptual errors may often arise. We will close this very brief general discussion of perception by referring to some of the most common types of perceptual errors which occur in human behaviour.

Errors of Perception

We have seen that the process of perception does not simply consist of the brain passively registering the information conveyed to it by the senses. What we actually perceive of any external event will depend not only on the event itself, but also on our past experiences and present anticipations. We cannot always believe the evidence of our own senses! Things are not always what they seem! In this section we will consider briefly how the perceiving individual reacts to situations where the sensory information is artificially distorted to produce illusory effects. An illusion may be defined as a false perception which occurs when our experience of the stimulus fails to correspond with the stimulus as it really is. Possibly one of the most commonly presented forms of visual illusion is the so-called 'Muller-Lyer' illusion where two lines of equal length are made to appear of different lengths by being bounded by arrows, as illustrated in Figure 7.

Figure 7

Line A is perceived as being shorter than line B due to the effect of the arrows.

Although the two lines are equal in length, line B appears longer than line A. Looking at the above lines it is virtually impossible to avoid seeing line B as longer than line A, in spite of the fact that we know the lines have been drawn of equal length. In seeking to understand why such an illusion occurs, we might notice that the ingoing arrows bounding line A correspond to the image received by the eye of the outside corner of a building or a box. The outgoing arrows on line B give the contrasting impression of the inside corner of a room. If these lines were part of three-dimensional forms such as buildings, we would quite rightly perceive the figure represented by line A as being nearer to us in space than that represented by line B. This incorporation of cues normally used for gauging distance into our perception of flat lines upsets the normal accuracy of our visual perception and predisposes us to see the lines as being unequal in length. It is then not surprising that this particularly illusory effect is found less in young as compared to older children. The young child has not yet had sufficient perceptual experience and is thus less easily misled by the factors which produce the optical illusion in the Muller-Lyer lines. Some psychologists have devised experimental demonstrations of visual illusions which are more complex in their effects and more dramatic in their presentation. One of the best known of these demonstrations is that produced by Ames and his colleagues (1953) by their construction of a 'distorted room'.

We all spend a great deal of our life within the confines of rooms. Although rooms may vary greatly in size and shape, they have certain characteristics in common. Thus the floor and ceiling are normally horizontal, the walls vertical and at right angles to each other. Ames and his colleagues constructed a room with trapezoidal floors and walls, where the right wall was smaller than the left and the normal rectangular convention of a room is ignored. When subjects are asked to view the room from outside, by means of a small window or peephole, they find themselves perceiving things which are quite contrary to common everyday experience. Thus, as Figure 8 demonstrates, three men who are of equal size are seen to vary strikingly in height so that the man on the left is seen as a midget and the man on the extreme right as a giant.

Figure 8

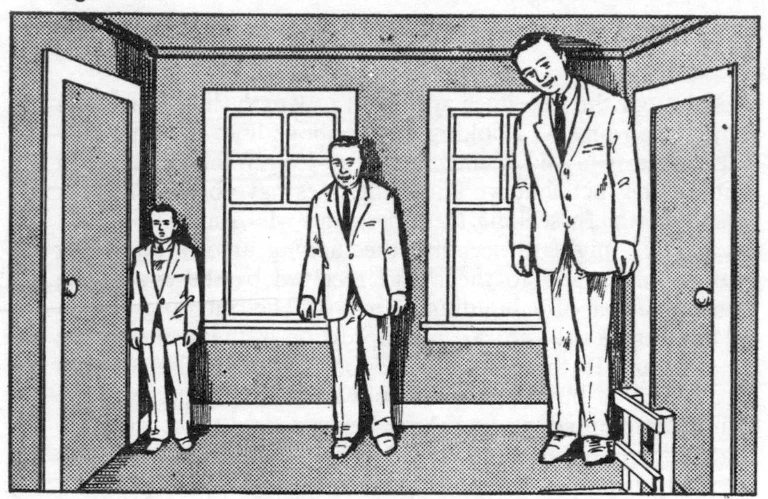

In actual fact, because of the distorted construction of the room, the man on the left is nearly twice as far away from the viewer as the man on the right. Using similar methods, Ames and his colleagues are able to produce a number of odd effects where, for example, balls appear to be rolling uphill or gradually changing in size. The effect of this illusion depends mainly on the fact that our past experience with rooms leads us to assume that the room is of a normal type. Once we do this, the people or objects in the room are seen in a distorted manner so as to correspond with our preconceptions regarding the room.

This experiment demonstrates that perceptual habits which help us to respond quickly and effectively to our normal environment may lead us to distort reality when our environment is changed in an unusual or unexpected manner. Some psychologists (Wittreich *et al.*, 1959) have demonstrated that other factors may influence the individual's response to the Ames room. Quite accidentally, Wittreich found that the distorted view of people as seen by viewers outside the Ames room may also vary according to the degree and type of emotional relationship between the viewer and the person perceived inside the room. Thus if one of the persons perceived inside the room has an emotional relationship with the outside viewer, this person tends to be seen in a less distorted way. Wittreich also found that if the person being viewed in the room was made to seem as if already distorted in some way (*e.g.* amputation of a limb), the normal distortion produced by the room was greatly lessened. It would appear that the errors of perception produced in this situation may depend not only on the present visual cues and past experience, but also on interpersonal factors.

Other psychologists have used a simpler devise to produce equally startling demonstrations of what happens when the visual information reaching the senses is other than that to which we are accustomed. Kohler (1961) asked volunteer subjects to wear special spectacles in which the normal retinal image was inverted. The effect of wearing such spectacles at first is to produce chaos and confusion in the subject, who finds himself living in a world in which everything appears upside down. One immediate effect of such visual distortion is for even simple movements to become awkward and difficult to execute. It is only very gradually that the subject becomes able to find his way about without feeling dizzy or bumping into objects. After a few days of constantly wearing the spectacles, Kohler's subjects reported that the world was beginning to switch back, from being upside down, to a normal orientation. Gradually the subjects began to see everything in the external world as being normally orientated and could even carry out such complex actions as riding a bicycle, although still wearing the inverted spectacles. The last stage of this experiment is perhaps the strangest. Here the subjects finally removed the spectacles and now found themselves perceiving everything upside down, although their senses were now receiving the normal retinal image. Kohler and his colleagues have carried out further experiments using different types of distorting spectacles with similar results. Thus, when the information conveyed to us by our senses is distorted from its habitual form, we are for a short time thrown off balance. Our brain soon learns however to recode such distorted information so as to allow the individual to behave in his habitual way in an abnormal sensory environment. Indeed, we adjust so well to the new environmental situation that when we are again exposed to our normal sensory environment there is a time lag before we are able to readapt in our mode of perception.

We have earlier observed that the way in which we perceive the outside world may be greatly affected by our current state of mind. If, for example, we are feeling particularly anxious, we will tend to perceive things rather differently than if we are quite relaxed. A number of recent studies of perception have indicated that the way we see things may be influenced not only by transient changes in mood, but also by more enduring attitudes which are a permanent part of our personality structure. The relationship between personality characteristics and perception has been the subject of a vast number of investigations which could not be described within the framework of the present book. The work of Witkin and his colleagues (1954) is illustrative of such investigations which demonstrate to what extent our feelings affect how we view the external world. Witkin used a wide range of experiments, the common element of which was that in each case the individual was required to attend selectively to visual stimuli while ignoring the influence of a changing background of stimulation. He found that some people showed a constantly passive perceptual attitude in that they were very easily influenced by background activity which disrupted their perception of an object in the foreground. Such subjects (termed 'field dependent' by Witkin) tended to be lacking in confidence, to be more anxious, to have less control over their feelings, and to be generally more passive and conforming in their attitude to authority. Other subjects, whose perceptual activity was less influenced by background activity ('field independent'), had the opposite type of personality. They tended to be more self-controlled, more assertive and self-confident and less anxious. Witkin and his colleagues were also able to show that 'field dependence' was typical of the perceptual attitude of the very young child who, however, tends to become progressively more independent and less easily influenced in his perception of the external world. It would thus seem that our level of emotional maturity is an important factor in influencing the way in which we perceive sensory data.

In discussing errors of perception we have thus far considered illusory experiences which consist of a misinterpretation of an existing stimulus. A distinction is often made between this type of perceptual error and an *hallucination* where perception occurs in the absence of any objective stimulus. Although it is customary to associate hallucination with the more serious forms of mental illness, such forms of experience are by no means limited to the psychotically disturbed patient. Many normal children are subject to hallucinatory experiences, such as in the case of the lonely child who invents an imaginary playmate who soon becomes as real to him as a true playmate. In certain states in adult life hallucinations can also occur. For example, lack of water and food, and fatigue can cause hallucinations such as are reported in mirages, and lack of oxygen in high altitudes has caused some pilots to experience hallucinations. Again, the hypnagogic state (the state of mind which exists just before we fall asleep) contains many types of normal hallucinations when our thoughts become images and are seen as actual events occurring in front of our eyes. We have already referred to our tendency to become hallucinated if we are deprived of the usual pattern of sensory stimulation. Any situation which blurs the individual's capacity to differentiate between inner sensation and outer events leads to a confused state where hallucinations may operate. Nurses will be familiar with the bizarre hallucinations often experienced by patients coming out of anaesthesia or while in a state of high fever. Some studies of hallucinatory activity make the point that emotionally disturbed people sometimes experience vivid visual and auditory hallucinations although they are not suffering from a psychotic illness. Perhaps the main distinction between these experiences and the hallucinations of the psychotic patient lies in the degree to which the patient accepts them as real events and allows them to control his behaviour. The insecure, rather hysterical person who is under severe emotional stress may report hearing voices or of seeing things that 'aren't there' but he usually has no difficulty in recognizing the difference between such an experience and a true perception. Sedman (1966) found that such 'pseudo-hallucinations' are reported much more frequently by females. When hallucinations do occur in a state of clear unclouded consciousness and are fully accepted by the patient as 'real' externally located events, it is likely that the patient is suffering from an affective or schizophrenic psychosis. Such 'pure' hallucinations may be seen to arise from a confusion between inner mental activity and outer events. The patient who cannot differentiate between his own thoughts and the voices of others who speak to him may experience some of his thoughts as coming from outside of him in the form of 'voices'. Other patients whose mental images become so real and confused with their perceptions of the outside world experience these images as 'real' events. We all make the same error in our dreams or in the hypnagogic state where we confuse inner thoughts and images with events occurring outside our bodies. It is little wonder that the psychotic patient has been referred to as 'a dreamer in a world awake'. It is often difficult to draw a clear distinction between an illusion and an hallucination. According to our definitions the main difference between these two forms of perceptual error is that an illusion is a misperception of an existing stimulus while an hallucination occurs without any stimulus. This distinction is apt to be misleading for hallucinations are too often set off by an internal or external stimulus. For example, a schizophrenic patient, who for various reasons was ignored both by her family and by patients and staff in the hospital, developed an hallucination of being surrounded by hundreds of children who kept her company. This hallucination was stimulated by the patient's loneliness and desire for human contact. As was the case with the illusory experiences earlier considered, hallucinations are all in varying degrees influenced by the current feeling and mental state of the individual.

Illness, particularly when it leads to hospital admission, is quite often an extremely traumatic experience for the individual. Apart from the anxiety induced by being ill, the patient is asked to adjust to the entirely new and unfamiliar environment of a hospital. To the nurse, who is well accustomed to the hospital environment, it is often difficult to put oneself in the place of the patient. To the patient, the hospital may represent an alien and frightening environment, full of sights and sounds that are new and unfamiliar. It takes time for him to reorientate himself to this new world, just as it once took the student nurse time to become used to her new surroundings. The patient's reactions to the hospital environment are of course intensified by the fact that, unlike the nurse, he has no specific role to play, his illness having placed him in the role of a passive participant. It is not surprising that patients are often easily upset and fearful during the first days in hospital and that they are likely to misinterpret or misperceive the strange happenings which are continually going on around them. An essential part of nursing care is in helping the patient to learn about his new environment, making the unfamiliar and frightening familiar and understandable, and wherever possible taking care to correct the patient's misperceptions. Part of the nurse's training is directed at improving her own perceptual attitudes in teaching her to look for and observe those aspects of the patient's behaviour that will be helpful to the diagnosis and general treatment of the patient while in hospital. Indeed, an essential quality of nursing is the gradual learning of new perceptual attitudes to people which help her to attend to features of behaviour that would hitherto have passed unnoticed. Perhaps one of the most difficult adjustments that the trainee nurse is required to make is to selectively perceive signs and symptoms which are relevant to the patient's illness, while at the same time retaining the capacity to perceive and react to the person behind the illness. To be a good observer and an efficient nurse, she must also learn that her feelings about individual patients may at times greatly influence and even distort her observations. We are all human, and it is unlikely that a nurse will find herself having a uniform reaction to all patients. She will find herself able to relate to some patients much more easily than to others. She will find some patients personally more likeable than others. Patients and nurses are people, and their reactions to each other will be governed by the same personal and emotional factors which come into play in any human relationship. In her professional role, however, the nurse must come to learn that her feelings about patients may greatly influence the accuracy and efficiency of her observations. She is required to make the very difficult adjustment between a spontaneous and warm interaction with the patient as a person, coupled with a certain degree of detachment in her response to the patient as a patient.

Concluding Remarks

Both attending and perceiving are active processes. We are not like cameras automatically transmitting data from the sense organs to the brain in a uniform pattern. Although our perception of events in the outside world usually corresponds to the actual events, it is equally true that no two people ever perceive the same event in *exactly* the same way. The act of perception calls into play the whole complex outlook of the individual. The fact that it is a person with his own unique outlook who is doing the perceiving means that there is a wide scope for perceptual errors, some of which we have considered here. As individuals, we all develop our own habitual ways of responding to events. These habits are a product of our personal experiences and together help to give us some degree of constancy and individuality. We have seen here that in some ways our perceptual response to our environment is a habitual process which may be highly resistant to change.

QUESTIONS

1. Discuss the *subjective* aspects of attending and perceiving. How does this subjective factor in perception affect our capacity to be accurate observers of events?

2. Describe the types of errors which may occur in normal perception. To what extent does knowledge of normal perceptual errors widen our understanding of the misperceptions made by patients while in hospital?

10. The Processes of Learning and Remembering

In the previous chapter we discussed the processes which enable us to become aware of our environment. If our environment has to have any lasting influence we must take the further step of learning the material which we have perceived. The degree to which learning has been effective is shown by our ability to retain the information learned and to recall it after a period of time. It is the capacities of learning and remembering which in fact allow us to accumulate the store of knowledge which we can selectively apply at a later date to deal with problems in our environment.

The Nature of Learning

When faced with such a difficult problem as understanding the many factors involved in human learning, psychologists began by studying the more simple problem of animal learning in controlled situations. It was found that most animals, when placed in a situation which demanded a certain amount of learning for the problem to be solved, behaved in a characteristic way. Thus a cat, for example, when placed in a cage which requires the manipulation of a certain lever to allow the animal to escape from the cage and to reach food placed outside, will behave first in an apparently random purposeless way. It will try to force itself out through the cage to reach the food and then it may begin to run round the cage, jumping up occasionally in an attempt to force a way out. Sooner or later its behaviour will result in it pressing the correct lever, apparently by accident, and the animal will escape. Placed in the same situation again the following day, the animal will behave in the same way although there will be a decreased amount of random behaviour before it touches the correct lever and thus solves the problem. Each time this experience is repeated there is a gradual reduction of errors and a shorter space of time elapsing before the animal gives the correct response to solve the problem. This form of learning is applicable to most problems which animals have to solve and we can say that the animal learns by carrying out a number of trials during which errors are gradually modified and corrected. In fact, this type of learning is known as *trial and error learning*.

Obviously human learning does not proceed in the same random manner. The solving of a problem in human learning is usually accompanied by a realization of the way in which the solution is achieved, a 'Now, I've got it!' feeling. When learning involves a sudden awareness of the method of solution we speak of *insightful learning* to distinguish it from the blinder manipulations of trial and error learning. If we examine the point of insight in human learning we find that it is composed of a repatterning of the elements of the learning situation. The subject suddenly perceives a new relationship between different parts of the problem which immediately leads to the solution. Insightful learning also means that, once the principle of solving the problem is solved, the subject has sufficient understanding of this principle to be able to apply it to other learning situations of the same type. A closer look at the human learning process, however, demonstrates that insight is usually achieved only after a great deal of trial and error. If we give a human subject a complicated and unfamiliar puzzle to solve he will invariably begin, like the animal, to try out various leads, gradually discarding the irrelevant ones. He will, in fact, learn by his errors to reduce the possible approaches to the problem until he is able to concentrate upon a few possibilities that appear to offer some hope of a solution. He may then suddenly perceive the correct method of attack out of the limited alternatives he has left. This final perception represents the point of insight at which all irrelevancies are discarded and the correct principle applied. If later faced with a similar type of problem the individual will be able to apply his previously acquired insight to find the solution without delay. The insight is, however, only achieved after an initial period of trial and error. In fact there will be several points of insight, each preceded by trial and error, where the subject comes nearer to the solution. Most learning performances proceed irregularly with sudden spurts which represent points where the learner has been able to reconstruct the situation to see it in a new way, making his performance more efficient. A person learning to type, for example, will soon reach a point where no further improvement in speed occurs. If learning has to proceed the typist must be able to see her task in a new way by eliminating inefficient work habits. This will bring about a higher level of performance until once again further improvement will depend upon new insight. A similar example can be seen in the case of the student nurse who learns her physiology lectures as work divorced from actual experience. Later she may see how the various facts she is learning fit together in the functioning of the human body. Finally, she will be able to relate these facts to increase her understanding of the patients' reactions to illness. Each of these insights will be accompanied by a higher level of her learning performance. The amount of trial and error compared with insightful learning which occurs will depend a great deal upon the type of learning situation. If the material to be learned is presented in such a way as to encourage only a passive attitude of amassing facts the possibilities of real insight will be decreased.

A third form of learning is represented by the process of *conditioning*. The influence of the conditioning process in learning was first demonstrated by a Russian physiologist, Pavlov, and in recent years has become one of the most important principles in the psychology of learning. A response is said to be conditioned when it is aroused by some stimulus other than the one which originally aroused it. For example, an animal such as a dog secretes saliva in its mouth at the sight of food. The secretion of saliva is the natural response and the food the unconditioned stimulus. If, however, a bell is rung on each occasion on which food is presented, the animal will learn to produce the salivary response towards the new stimulus of the bell even when the food is not present. The bell has now become the conditioning stimulus and the saliva response may be said to have been conditioned.

This form of conditioning, in which unconditioned responses are linked with a new range of stimuli, is often called *Classical Conditioning* to distinguish it from *Operant Conditioning*. This latter form of conditioning is a much more active form of learning in which certain responses are strengthened by *reinforcement*. If we put a hungry animal in a cage it will prowl around looking for food. Let us say we have arranged things so that a meat pellet will drop into the cage when a particular lever is pressed. If the lever is accidentally pressed by the animal and the food duly delivered, the animal will soon learn to press the lever to obtain further food. The reward of food thus *reinforces* the lever-pressing response. We might now decide to make the learning situation a little more complex by reinforcing the lever-pressing only when the response is emitted while a light in the cage is on. Soon we will have conditioned the animal to press the lever only when the light is shining. We might next begin to reinforce the animal when he presses the bar with his *left* paw and while the light is on. We could go on to condition the animal into performing a range of fairly complex actions by 'stamping in' certain actions at the expense of others. Indeed, this is exactly the procedure the animal trainer might adopt in order to teach his circus animals new tricks. However, any habit which has been learned may be unlearned, and this will happen if we later forget to continue rewarding the animal when the trick is performed correctly. The omission of reinforcement would soon lead to the *extinction* of the learned pattern of behaviour. Studies of operant conditioning indicate however that reinforcement need not occur every time the correct response is made. The habit will continue to operate if it is reinforced only part of the time.

Although the application of classical conditioning to human behaviour is limited, no such restriction applies in the case of operant conditioning. A great deal of child rearing, for example, may be seen as a series of operant conditioning situations. With a child there is of course no necessity to reward desirable behaviour with food, although often sweets may take the place of meat pellets. Parents constantly condition their child's conduct by reinforcing, with some verbal or non-verbal sign of approval, those aspects of his behaviour which they wish to encourage. Reinforcement need not of course always take a positive form. Parental disapproval, conveyed by word or direct action, conditions the child to continually inhibit certain actions because they have now become associated with displeasure. In conditioned learning of this type the individual may be entirely unaware that his behaviour is being influenced. Verplanck (1955) demonstrated how the verbal behaviour of college students could be altered by applying operant conditioning techniques to their spontaneous speech. In a series of informal conversations with the students, Verplanck reinforced by nods and other signs of approval all statements of opinion beginning with phrases like 'I think . . .', 'I believe . . .', and so on. By the end of the experiment the frequency of such statements in the students' speech had greatly increased. In another study (Azrin and

Lindsley, 1956) operant conditioning was successfully applied to increase co-operative behaviour between a group of children at play. In neither of these experiments had the subjects any idea that their behaviour was being conditioned. It may be argued that a great many of our individual characteristics of behaviour, our adult preferences and aversions, may be due to past conditioning experiences. Specific fears may be learned in a similar manner. Many years ago, Watson (1920) demonstrated how a child's fear of furry animals might be conditioned by producing a frighteningly loud noise each time a child was playing with a hitherto loved furry toy.

Later, Jones (1924) illustrated how a similar phobia could be alleviated by applying the laws of conditioning in reverse to decondition the child's fear response. This aspect of conditioning brings us to the possible application of conditioned learning to the understanding of emotional disturbance. During Pavlov's experiments some of the animals were almost drowned when the room in which their cage stood was flooded with water. Thereafter, the sight of water in any form produced an instant reaction of panic in these animals. The original response of panic to the fear of being drowned had now in fact become conditioned to the stimulus of water in any form. We can compare this situation to, let us say, a child who is bitten by a dog when walking under a tunnel. In later life he might develop a fear of enclosed spaces and we might explain this on the basis that his original fear at being attacked by the dog had now become conditioned to the other stimulus present at the time, namely, the enclosed space of the tunnel. In recent years the concept of conditioning has been applied to the treatment of behaviour disorders. Treatment according to this method consists of an attempt to 'decondition' the behaviour in question. The childhood behaviour 'disorders' of enuresis and nail-biting provide examples of such deconditioning methods. The enuretic child is made to sleep on a mat which is connected to electrodes. If he wets the bed this automatically produces a short circuit in the system and a bell rings. The child is made to rise and go to the bathroom at the sound of the bell on all occasions. Repeated experiences such as this lead, it is hoped, to the child being conditioned to respond to his bladder tensions rather than the bell. This technique is based on one of the principles of modern learning theory, that of 'reciprocal inhibition' which aims at disrupting an unwanted habit pattern by introducing a new response which is incompatible with the response which is to be extinguished.

This represents but one example of the application of learning theory to the modification of human behaviour. Another principle of learning theory, that of 'satiation' holds that repeated voluntary practice of a habit in the absence of the force motivating the habit will again result in its gradual extinction.

Thus children who are habitual nail-biters may be treated by being made to bite their nails on schedule. the idea being that repetition of nail-biting at times when the inner tension normally producing it is absent will lead to a falling off of the habit. Patients with uncontrollable facial tics have again been treated in this way by having them reproduce the tic in front of a mirror over planned practice periods. This approach to the problem regards neurotic behavioural habits as learned patterns of behaviour which can be understood and treated by the application of normal learning theory. It is in flat contradiction to the dynamic approach of psychoanalysis which would regard the neurotic habit as being only a symptom of underlying mental conflict. Our extinction of the neurotic habit, be it nail-biting, enuresis or facial tic, would then merely remove the individual's means of expressing his problem while leaving the problem itself untouched. The obvious answer would seem to lie in the future behaviour of the patient after treatment. If the learning theory argument is correct the patient should literally be cured while, according to the alternative argument, one would expect the later appearance of new symptoms in expression of the patient's untreated and unconscious conflicts. Reports by those who practise 'behaviour therapy,' as those conditioning procedures have come to be known, are emphatic that subsequent breakdown is an infrequent occurrence after treatment. Follow-up studies in this field are, however, few and open to criticism on many grounds so the issue is still open. What does appear to be certain is that the application of learning theory to neurotic disorders and their treatment might lead to a fuller appreciation of the many little-understood processes which occur in all forms of psychotherapy.

Learning and the Physiological Limit

A person's learning performance may be continually improved as new insights are gained and inefficient learning habits rejected. There comes a time, however, when the learning performance appears to reach a maximum level where there is no possibility of further improvement. If the learning task involves physical effort we might consider that the person had reached the limit of their physical capacity. If the task is a mental one we might say that the person has reached their maximum mental level. The maximum learning performance of which the individual is capable is termed the *physiological limit* which is a function of the mental and physical constitution of the individual. It has been experimentally demonstrated that most people function at a level well below their physiological limit. Most of us are content to jog along at a rate which; although not inefficient, is well below the maximum effort of which we are capable. We may, in fact, be passed by others who, although of lower ability, have the forcefulness and drive to work at their maximum level. Apart from this conscious lack of effort there would also seem to be another, less consciously operating, factor which prevents us reaching our true work limits. This can be demonstrated quite simply by an apparatus called an 'ergograph'. This machine sets the subject the task of raising different weights with one finger. After a short time the subject's pull becomes weaker until he reaches the point where he feels that his finger is exhausted. If he is given a further incentive, like money, or that provided by competing with a fellow subject, he may find that he can continue with the task for another period. Even when incentives no longer have any effect and muscular fatigue appears to have set in, the subject may again continue if told (incorrectly) that a lighter weight is being substituted for the present one. In fact, the apparent physiological limit of the individual is seldom reached, the maximum level of performance being controlled by a *psychological limit*. This fact is well illustrated by the now almost commonplace achievement of the four-minute mile in athletics. For many years it was considered that the time limit of four minutes represented an insuperable barrier to the physiological capabilities of the athlete. Roger Bannister and his trainer, however, regarded this barrier as a psychological one which could be overcome not only with physical effort but with the correct psychological attitude. Their view was confirmed not only by Bannister's triumph but by the fact that, once the barrier had been crashed, many other athletes were able to follow in his footsteps. There is no doubt that the same logic can be applied to purely mental effort. Too often people are prevented from giving of their best, not because they are not capable, but because they set their aspirations well below their capabilities. If the psychological attitude to the learning situation is wrong it will forever act as a brake on future achievement.

Those who rise to the top of their tree often do so by virtue of their self-confident freedom from such self-imposed restrictions. We have already said that maturity involves a recognition and acceptance of one's own limitations but we cannot hope to know our limitations without testing ourselves. It is a true adage that we never know what we are capable of until we try.

The reference here to self-confidence brings up another interesting point on fatigue. Studies of the effects of fatigue in different practical learning situations show that, during the initial period of fatigue, the subject is invariably unaware of the effects of the fatigue on his performance which he considers to be as accurate as before. Later, when fatigue becomes more pronounced, he recognizes its implications and may then make allowances for its effect upon his performance. Such information is of great practical value in industry and other fields where accuracy of performance is essential. It requires little imagination to apply the same facts to the nurse's role and to see the dangers of slight and moderate degrees of fatigue in this setting. The nurse who is very tired will probably recognize this and avoid any aspect of her work which demands extreme accuracy at that time. If, however, she is only slightly tired she may overlook its effects on the accuracy of her work with dangerous results. These facts also provide a telling argument against the twelve-hour shift system. Our consideration of the psychological limit also reminds us that fatigue may at times be a psychological reaction of the nurse to her duties. Nurses become more quickly tired in wards where the atmosphere is not conducive to high staff morale. We have earlier remarked on the dangerous influence of boredom on accurate work, although the reader may reflect that this is becoming an increasingly unlikely occurrence in the complex course of the present-day nurse's duties.

Motivation in Learning

In considering fatigue we have already introduced the role of motivation in learning. People do not learn efficiently without purpose. Real learning will occur only in the presence of an effective incentive. Applying this to nursing training we might say that, no matter how well the lectures and general training are presented, the nurse will not learn effectively unless she is stimulated to do so by an incentive. This incentive may be financial, it may take the form of competition with one's fellow students, or, more desirably, it may simply be a pride of succeeding in one's job. The incentive may include these and many other aspects but it must be present in some form. Thus far we have been considering the learner as an isolated subject but the recognition of the influence of motivation reminds us that there can be no learner without a teacher. Directly connected with motivation in the learning situation is the important factor of *identification*. We have already referred to the process of identification in dealing with the personality defence mechanisms and here we are only interested in its bearing upon learning. The effect of identification on learning is, of course, seen most clearly in the increase in the range of the young child's activities which occurs through identification with the parent. The opposite type of situation is illustrated by the child who develops a positive aversion to some of his school subjects because of his dislike of the master who teaches them. The principle could be broadly stated to the effect that learning may be facilitated or inhibited according to the type of relationship existing between the teacher and the learner. This is particularly true in relation to the adolescent student nurse who is apt to identify herself with her seniors. It is then a responsibility of the teacher, whether she is the class tutor or ward sister, to be a worthy person who will act as a suitable model for the young nurse. We will return to consider the teacher's role in the next section but, before leaving the influence of identification on the learning process, it is worth noting that the nurse might also function as a source of identification for the patient. This is particularly true in mental nursing where the nurse-patient relationship provides an intimate learning situation. In his relations with the nurse the mental patient learns to modify his habits and ways of thinking in accordance with the personality of the nurse. The most chronic and severely ill (psychotic) the patient is the more this principle applies. The author was some time ago involved in a rehabilitation scheme for chronic psychotic patients and in their appraisal of the success of the scheme he and his colleagues had this to say: 'We conclude that the physical material in the environment, while useful, was not the most important factor in producing the change (in the patients). It was the nurses; and the most important thing about the nurses and other people in their environment, is how they feel about their patients . . .' (Cameron, Laing, McGhie, 1955). As already emphasized, the nurse also learns nursing from her patients and the value of identification will therefore be increased if the identification is a reciprocal process. The most effective nurse can put herself in the patient's place and thus gain some understanding of the patient's feelings.

Learning and Education

It may seem rather naïve to ask what is the purpose of learning but this question is more relevant than we might at first think. Learning is the process of education so let us first consider the functions and general aim of education. Education has often been compared to the following analogy: 'The contents of a jug have to be transferred to a bottle with a narrow neck. If we pour carefully and steadily most of the fluid will reach the bottle, although some of it may be spilled. At the end of the process the bottle will contain the previous contents of the jug.' If we replace the jug with the material to be learned, the bottle with the learner and regard the teacher as the one who does the pouring we have the traditional view of education. In this form education simply means the transmission of information from teacher to learner. If, however, we consult a dictionary we find that to educate meant originally 'to bring out, develop, from latent or potential existence'. In this sense the function of education is to create a stimulating background which will stimulate the students to realize their own personalities and to think for themselves.

Let us first take a closer look at our 'jug and bottle' conception of learning. In this analogy the bottle will gradually come to contain the same fluid as is poured out of the jug. In other words, it is assumed that the teacher's knowledge will be transmitted directly to the learner who will assimilate it in a passive way. Human learning is, however, essentially an active process and knowledge is never transmitted in this direct and passive way. Earlier we explained the fact that each individual perceives what goes on in his environment in his own unique way. Each person, in fact, brings to the educational setting his own individual outlook and assumptions based upon previous experiences. If we refer this to the classroom setting we can deduce that each student may interpret the material given in a distinct and individual way. In other words, communication is never direct but depends upon the background of experience of those involved. One of the chief problems in the education of children is that the adult educator often assumes that his and the child's view of the world are comparable. A friend recently told me of an amusing incident which beautifully expressed the error of such an assumption. He was visiting a home where the mother was telling him how her little boy loved Sunday School which he had just started to attend. While my friend was in the home the little lad returned from Sunday School with eyes aglow and obviously very excited. When asked how he had enjoyed this week's session the child replied: 'Mummy, it was terribly exciting today!' The mother smiled at this confirmation of the boy's interest in Sunday School. She then asked her son what had made it so exciting and was rather shaken by the child's reply: 'Oh, Mummy, a wee boy escaped!' The same error is often made in adult education in that it is assumed that material taught will mean the same to each student. Teachers soon see the results of this erroneous assumption when they come to read over examination papers and are bewildered by the variety of ways in which students have interpreted their lectures. It is easy to adopt the defensive attitude that misinterpretation implies stupidity or inattention on the part of the students and to forget that the teacher's job is to ensure that what he says is understood by all. By encouraging the students to ask questions at the end of the lecture the teacher may be able to correct some misapprehensions and fill in some of the gaps in the students' understanding. It is, however, very difficult to formulate questions correctly if one has not already a good grasp of the subject. The silence which follows 'Any questions?' often denotes complete bewilderment rather than complete understanding.

This view of education as a passive transmission of knowledge is directly connected with equally outmoded didactic methods of teaching. Didactic teaching is essentially the traditional classroom lecture method where the students' only task is to ensure that they stay awake during the lecture. It has been said, with some truth, that no man learns from the experience of others and this is certainly one of the main disadvantages of traditional methods of teaching. Learning, if it is to be effective at all, must be active and we might contrast didactic learning with *participation learning* which involves both teacher and learner in active co-operation. Modern educational methods are based upon this concept of learning where the emphasis is on discussion rather than direct instruction. Most learning occurs in a group situation and this fact may be utilized in participation learning. By group discussion the students are able to exchange their ideas and learn from the views of others. By comparing their knowledge of their subject with that of their fellow students they are able to correct their false assumptions and misapprehensions. The teacher's role in such a setting is that of the group leader who supplies information where necessary and ensures that each member of the group is allowed ample opportunity to participate in the process. This avoids the dangers of the passive type of 'rote learning' where the student merely drinks in information which will be regurgitated later upon an examination paper. Learning becomes instead meaningful and insightful, thus invigorating an experience which is too often static and impersonal. What is learned must also be later applied in practice. Material which is learned in theory alone is liable to remain academic and sterile. Participation learning allows the student ample opportunity to put theory into practice.

These principles have been well incorporated into nursing training in recent years. The General Nursing Council now stress the need for active meaningful learning in the nurses' training. Emphasis is placed upon the need to integrate the various subjects which the nurse learns so that they become inter-related. Anatomy, physiology, neurology, etc., are but different approaches to the same general subject, the 'functioning of the human individual'. As a psychologist one cannot help but feel encouraged by the recent inclusion of psychology as another link in this chain of understanding. Today there is also much more awareness of the need for co-operation between the different authorities—particularly the doctor, the tutor, and the ward sister—who are responsible for the nurses' training. More recognition is being especially directed to the all-important role of the supervisory nurse as a focus of teaching. The same educational advances are taking place in mental nursing since the publication of the World Health Organization Report on the role of the mental nurse (*W.H.O. Report*, 1957). Mental nursing has tended to be regarded hitherto as a poor relation of general nursing. Recent developments in the orientation of nursing are, however, bound to affect the future status of mental nursing. In a series of papers reviewing the role of the mental nurse the present author expressed the opinion that '. . . recent years have seen a growing infiltration of the principles of mental nursing into general nursing, and basic general nursing programmes are being increasingly designed to include attention to mental health and the understanding of human relationships as intrinsic features of all nursing' (McGhie, 1957).

Let us now return to our opening question regarding the true aim of education. We might now answer this question by saying that education aims at widening a person's understanding of the world about him. It does this, not merely by acquainting people with new facts, but by aiding them to be less rigid in their assumptions and their way of thinking. It encourages them to develop their own personality by freeing them from the restriction of ignorance. It thus draws out of a person what is latent within him by encouraging him to think for himself. Education which aims merely at the transmission of information is limited and will tend only to discourage true learning with insight.

We have already stressed the necessity for learning to be related to practice. At times, however, this relationship will be an indirect and general one. From time to time I have been asked by nurses what relevance certain topics in my lectures have to their work. My reply is simply that any knowledge which widens our understanding of human behaviour must ultimately affect our efficiency both as a worker and as a person. If we close our minds to any educational influences which do not appear to have an immediate and direct bearing on our present tasks we merely succeed in becoming 'narrow-minded' and limited personalities.

The Nurse as a Behaviour Modifier

Earlier in this chapter, we referred to the application of conditioning procedures to the modification of human behaviour. In recent years, such forms of behaviour modification have expanded greatly and have been applied with considerable success in widely diverse settings. One important factor common to most forms of behaviour modification is that the best agents to institute the desired behavioural changes are often the people who have the most frequent contact with the individual concerned. Such people have more opportunity to observe the day-to-day behaviour of the individual and are in the best position to influence his behaviour. Thus, teachers are obviously the most suitable personnel to apply procedures designed to modify the classroom behaviour of their pupils. It seems equally clear that, if the proposed modification refers to the behaviour of patients in hospital, the therapeutic agent of choice is the nurse who is in constant contact with the patients.

Thus far, the majority of attempts to involve nursing personnel in behavioural modification techniques have been restricted to nurses working with psychiatric or mentally retarded patients. The main reason for the concentration of behavioural techniques on these populations is simply that it is often the maintenance of specific deviant behaviours which prevents such patients being accepted by the community outside of hospital. Thus, many chronically psychotic individuals manage to function outside of hospital because their deviant behaviours are not of the type to alarm others. To put it rather crudely, if an individual quietly hallucinates to himself, this behaviour may go comparatively unnoticed. If, however, he shrieks back loudly at his persecuting voices, his aberrant behaviour is more evident and likely to disturb others. Some years ago, I was involved in the treatment of an elderly psychotic lady who had frequent visual and auditory hallucinations of being in contact with God and other biblical figures. She was extremely vocal about such experiences and insisted on relating them in detail to everyone she met. As a result, people began to avoid her socially, struck her off as a suitable baby-sitter and turned her into a social isolate. Treatment in hospital helped to eradicate a number of other deviant symptoms she had developed but left her vivid, hallucinating experiences unabated. Finally, we persuaded her to agree not to communicate such experiences to others for a period of one month after discharge from hospital. During this period, she found that neighbours and friends were a great deal more accepting of her and that, accordingly, life was more pleasant. Such rewards made her more ready to continue this maintenance of privacy regarding her hallucinatory experiences and she was gradually reinstated in her community. This is a very simple illustration of the manner in which the modification of one aspect of behaviour may bring considerable positive benefits to the person concerned.

One of the best illustrations of the potentialities of nursing staff as behaviour therapists of psychiatric patients is contained in the study of Ayllon and Michael (1959) which sees the nurse as a 'behavioural engineer'. Implicit in this rather awkward sounding term is the notion that, as the 'tender loving care' spontaneously given by nurses is one of the most rewarding set of stimuli in the lives of chronic patients, it makes good sense to consciously harness and direct this as a therapeutic agent to normalize patient behaviour. A further related point is that the sympathy and concern shown by nurses to their patients, if not sensibly directed, may have the effect of maintaining the aberrant behaviours which keep the patient in hospital.

One study, carried out in a large psychiatric hospital in Canada, trained the nursing staff as prime therapists in modifying some of the most persistent and socially unacceptable behaviours shown by their chronic psychotic or retarded patients. Nurses were initially given training in methods of objectively recording the frequency of such specific behaviours and noting the events which appeared to stimulate such behaviours and reinforce their continuance. Next, the nurses were instructed on appropriate behavioural strategies which might be expected to reduce the frequency of such behaviours. After a period of altering the patients' social environment accordingly, the nurses re-evaluated the occurrence of such behaviours to assess the efficacy of their intervention. The results of this programme were dramatically effective and acted as a powerful reinforcement to the nursing staff's new behavioural role.

Let us briefly consider one or two typical examples of the types of problems which were successfully tackled in this way.

One female psychotic patient talked incessantly of her bizarre delusional beliefs. The frequency and volubility of her psychotic speech commanded a great deal of nursing attention, either because the nurse thought that her listening might give her insight into the patient's problems, or more often because she simply did not wish to be impolite by totally ignoring the verbal barrage. Other patients were less patient and frequently reacted with verbal or physical abuse towards their offending companion. The nurses in the ward were taught to keep a record of the frequency and length of these outbursts of delusional speech for five days before treatment was commenced. Subsequent treatment simply consisted of having the nurses politely but firmly withdraw their attention from the delusional speech while giving more of their time, attention and interest to the patient's less frequent periods of 'normal' speech. This simple procedure led to a dramatic decrease in the patient's psychotic speech and in the amount of aggressive behaviour aimed at the patient by her fellow patients. It is of interest to note that the undoubted success of this intervention was sporadically interrupted by other staff who felt sorry for the patient and listened sympathetically to her outbursts. Their undoubtedly well meaning actions only reinforced the undesirable behaviours and delayed the ultimate effectiveness of the treatment procedure.

Another chronic patient would never eat unless spoon-fed. It was noticed that this patient was also very fastidious about her appearance and dress and this fact was seized on as an integral part of a programme aimed at modifying her eating behaviour. Nurses were instructed to continue spoon-feeding but to do this in an increasingly careless fashion. As a result the patient's clothing would be stained with food after each meal. A'ter 12 days of this regime the patient began to feed herself with a resultant weight gain of over 20 lbs.

Another patient in the same study demonstrated chronic hoarding of ward towels. Each day she collected all available towels in the ward and hoarded them in her room. Here the behavioural intervention was based upon the principle of satiation. Nursing staff discontinued removing towels from her room and instead delivered an increasing number of towels to the patient's room each day. By the third week of the satiation procedure 60 towels were being delivered per day and the patient could hardly move around her room for piles of towels. Soon the patient began to remove the towels from her room faster than they were being replaced. At this point, where towel collecting had become aversive to the patient, the staff ceased their deliveries. The patient cleared her room of all but her own towels and a one year follow-up showed no reappearance of this aberrant behaviour.

Many studies have demonstrated the usefulness of 'token economy programmes' in modifying the behaviour of chronic psychiatric or retarded patients in more normal directions. Usually the procedure is to reward patients with tokens for such desirable behaviours as grooming themselves, non-aggressive behaviour, working around the ward, and so on. The tokens may be used to purchase a number of amenities such as cigarettes, confectioneries, late night T.V. watching, etc. Such programmes have been shown to be successful in increasing the incidence of various constructive behaviours and reducing the incidence of anti-social or destructive behaviours.

The illustrations already cited are mainly based upon the principle of positive reinforcement—rewarding desirable behaviour. Other forms of behaviour modification rely upon the principle of negative reinforcement or the punishment of undesirable behaviour. Such procedures are usually employed in attempting to modify behaviours which, although socially undesirable, give satisfaction to the individual. Thus, one treatment of adult child-molesters is to expose them to films or slides of children and present them with an aversive stimulus (e.g. electric shock) when the visual stimulus produces sexual arousal. Repeated experience of this situation results in the individual having aversive reactions to the stimulus (sexual thoughts of children) which once elicited positive responses. Although such aversive conditioning procedures may play an effective part in eradicating socially unacceptable behaviours, they usually require the complement of other more positively directed procedures. Thus, child-molesters so treated might also be given training in social skills aimed at increasing their competence in relating socially to adults of the opposite sex—this being an aspect of behaviour in which they usually have profound problems.

Most programmes of behaviour modification try to encourage the patient to be his own therapist by introducing an element of *self-control* into the treatment regime. Many people are not fully aware of the frequency with which they indulge in undesirable behaviours. Often, simply introducing them to simple techniques of self-observation greatly helps them to monitor and change their own behaviour. For example, if chronic insomniacs are taught to record their ways of reacting to their inability to sleep, they often come to appreciate that many of their habitual reactions only serve to reinforce their insomnia. Similarly, parents of hyperactive children have found that by monitoring their own reactions to their child's behaviour they became more aware of their own role in eliciting the hyperactive behaviours in their child.

Many of the strategies used in behaviour modification appear disconcertingly simple and at a common-sense level. However, they illustrate again that commonsense, correctly and continuously applied, may be surprisingly effective in changing human behaviour. While it would be a mistake to overestimate the power of such behavioural techniques and to see them as a universal panacea for all undesirable behaviours, it is equally erroneous to ignore their usefulness.

Readers who would wish a more thorough treatment of this topic than the very cursory reference contained herein might like to read one of the many relevant texts such as Kazdin's (1975) paperback, *Behaviour Modification in Applied Settings*.

The Process of Remembering

Although we discuss it separately, the process of memory cannot be divorced from that of learning. Many apparent forms of memory deficit are actually learning deficiencies for we cannot hope to recall something which has been inadequately learned. Adequate learning, in its turn, is partially dependent upon the earlier sequence of attention and perception, so that these factors all operate in the learning process. Remembering is in fact the final stage in the learning process by which we are able to make use of the stored-up results of previous learning. Although in recent years psychologists have reported many studies of human memory, there is still a great deal we do not fully understand. Like most of our human attributes we tend to take memory very much for granted, although without this capacity we would be less than human. If we were not able to store our previously learned knowledge and subsequently recall it when needed, everything presented to us would require to be learned anew. Apart from being an essential part of our general operating efficiency, the capacity of memory is also one of the basic factors in allowing us to develop and maintain our relationships with others. We cannot form an enduring relationship with anyone unless we are capable of recalling the existence of that person in his absence. We have already seen that the ability of the child to form a relationship with his mother, or with others around him, must await the gradual development of recall memory towards the latter end of the first year of life. In this chapter we shall confine ourselves to a very cursory examination of our present state of knowledge of some aspects of the memory process.

The Retention of Memories

We have as yet no direct way of knowing exactly where in the brain our memories are located or what form such records take. Neurological work indicates that the temporal lobes of the brain are vitally important for remembering, in that injury here has a profound effect on memory. Recent advances in biochemical analysis suggest that the retention of information induces changes in the structure of ribonucleic acid molecules contained in individual neurons, and a great deal of current research would appear to be taking us nearer to an understanding of the physiological correlates of memory. However, most of the findings at present are very tentative and for the present we rely mainly on psychological models of memory, based on the results of investigations of the way human beings handle information.

A long-accepted view of the retentive process is that the storage of newly learned material causes a structural change (a *memory trace*) somewhere in the brain. This theory then envisages each memory as having a fixed anatomical location, the multitude of memory traces constituting a permanent record of our previous experiences. Although this conception of a memory trace is far too simple to fit all known facts about human memory, it has some neurophysiological support. A Canadian neurosurgeon, Penfield (1954), demonstrated that memories may be reactivated by direct electrical stimulation of the temporal lobe of the cortex. Under such stimulation Penfield's patients reported experiencing memory images which were so clear, detailed, and vivid as to cause some of them to be confused with current events. Some of the memories evoked in this way were of events in the far distant past, having occurred in the early life of a now elderly person. Penfield was also able to show that the memories reproduced by patients in his experiments varied according to the part of the brain stimulated by the electrode. This work would appear to support the view that every memory is stored somewhere in the brain in the form of a structural change in the brain cells.

An alternative theory suggests that memories may consist of active patterns of electrical impulses which have no specific anatomical location. This view would regard memories as patterns of neural activity which do not involve any structural change. Although it would be extremely difficult to confirm directly such a theory of memory, there are indirect ways of assessing its validity. If memory exists in the form of electrical activity we would expect any event which greatly disturbs the electrical activity in the brain to have a profound effect on previously stored memories. One of the simplest ways of producing a gross disruption of the electrical activity in the brain is by massive electroshock or by freezing the brain and reducing the electrical activity to a minimum. For obvious reasons such experiments have been confined to animals. The animal is taught a new task and, after an interval, retested on the same task to see how much of the previous learning has been retained. At some time after the first learning performance electroconvulsive shock is introduced and the animal subsequently retested on the same task. The second performance thus gives some indication of the degree to which shock has affected the retentive process. At first glance is would seem that the results of such experiments go against the theory that memories consist of electrical activity, in that the shock does not produce any discernible effect on subsequent performance. However, much appears to depend on the length of time elapsing between the first learning experience and the disruptive effects of the shock treatment. In some experiments it was shown that electroconvulsive shock had no effect on the animal's performance if the shock was given fifteen minutes or more after the first learning experience. However, if the shock was given after a shorter post-learning interval, memory loss was apparent. Where the shock was given only a few minutes after the initial learning, memory loss was complete. These results suggest that memory is most vulnerable to disturbance within a short interval after learning, and that, once this critical period is passed, the memory becomes consolidated in the brain and highly resistant to further interference. Such findings suggest that both theories of storage may be correct and that there are two types of memories. This model indicates that information is initially held in a *short-term* storage system as a pattern of electrical activity. After a short time the information is transferred to a more stable *long-term* storage system, as a permanent change in the structure of the brain cells.

The Two-phase Theory of Memory

We have already indicated that there is some evidence to suggest that there may be two separate stages in the memory process. A useful, although over-simplified, psychological model of this process has been provided by Broadbent (1958) and is illustrated in Figure 9.

Figure 9

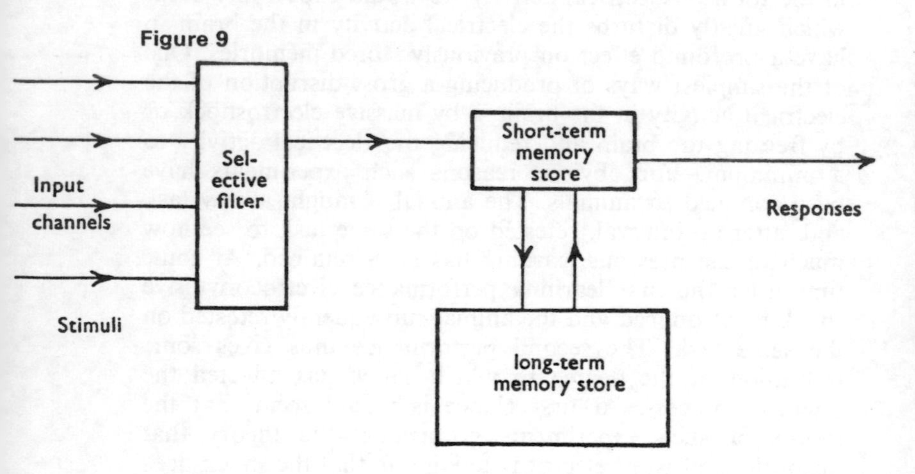

In considering attention, we have already seen that we can attend to only one source of stimulation at a time and that attention may then be regarded as a selective filtering of the sensory input from the environment. The information which is selectively attended to then passes into a short-term memory store where it may be held for a short time before being passed into the more permanent and stable long-term memory store. However, as it would be uneconomical for us to retain a permanent record of every event, information may be held in the short-term memory store only long enough to allow an appropriate response to be made. Thus we may wish to remember a telephone number only long enough to be able to dial it. In this case there would be no need to transfer the information to the more permanent long-term memory store. One advantage of such a two-phase model of memory lies in the fact that these two systems of storage appear to operate on somewhat different principles. Much recent work suggests that, when things go wrong during the memory process, the fault usually occurs during the initial phase of short-term memory storage.

Let us consider some of the differences between these two storage phases. Although our long-term memory appears to have an almost unlimited capacity for storing information, this is certainly not the case with short-term memory which is very restricted in the amount of information it can handle at any one time. Although it would be untrue to say that information once transferred to the long-term store is forever safe from interference, it does not seem to be much more durable and stable. Information being held in the short-term store, in contrast, is extremely susceptible to interference by the arrival of new information. If, for example, we are interrupted momentarily while dialling a telephone number by someone asking, say, a simple question, this may be sufficient to completely wipe out our memory of the required number sequence. In our day-to-day life we frequently have to hold in mind for a short time quite lengthy sequences of information which in their raw form would be too much for the restricted capacity of our short-term memory. To ease the load on short-term memory we may perform a kind of coding process on the incoming information. For example, if I am asked to remember the following number sequence—106658441007372436, this difficult task may become a great deal simpler if I am able to reduce the load by combining some of the numbers into easily remembered groups. The number in our example may be seen as composed of 1066 (the date of the Battle of Hastings), 58441 (which happens to be my telephone number), 007 (which need not be explained to the James Bond fan), finally leaving six numbers (37-24-36) which represents some interesting and well-known statistics. We are seldom asked to remember such a long number sequence, but in listening to someone speaking we perform almost exactly the same coding procedure in registering sequences of words as groups or phases, rather than as individual words. We are also aided by the fact that language contains a great many words which, although grammatically correct, are not strictly necessary for comprehension. When someone is speaking we need not burden our limited storage capacity with these redundant words which can be easily filled in later because they are determined by their context. The same idea can also be illustrated by the fact that most people find no difficulty in understanding a written passage in which half of the words (the more redundant ones) are missing. (A fact well known to those who compile newspaper headlines.)

In an earlier section we referred to the complaint of poor memory commonly made by elderly people. Studies of changes in memory with age suggest that such difficulties are nearly always located in the short-term phase of memory. As we grow older the amount of information which can be held in short-term memory at any one time appears to decrease and the effect of interference is greatly enhanced (Broadbent and Heron, 1962; Inglis, 1965; McGhie *et al.*, 1965). Some of the effects of normal ageing on short-term memory are also evident in an exaggerated form in patients with organic cerebral disease. Patients with a senile dementia show a pronounced breakdown in short-term memory storage which is often the first observable sign of their pathological condition. A similar type of memory deficit has been noted in some forms of schizophrenia (McGhie *et al.*, 1965 *a*, 1965 *b*). The relative failure of short-term retention in such patients helps to explain their obvious difficulty in concentrating and in communicating adequately with others. Severely subnormal defectives show a surprisingly good retention of information which has had time to be assimilated into long-term storage, whereas their short-term memory is poor. If groups of low-grade defectives and normals are compared in their ability to recall sequences of information after varying time intervals, it can be shown that in the defective group most of the forgetting occurs within two seconds following the presentation of the information (Hermelin and O'Connor, 1964). Other types of patients with severe memory disorder show very little impairment of short-term memory, but appear to have lost the ability to retain more permanent memories. For example, in Korsakow's psychosis, an organic disorder of the nervous system, the patient may retain events well enough for a short period, but be unable to form more lasting durable memories. In terms of Broadbent's model, we might interpret this as being due to a failure in the hypothetical mechanism which transfers information from short-term into long-term storage.

Failures in Recall (Forgetting)

We usually become interested in the memory process at the point where it breaks down or operates in a faulty fashion so we will now go on to consider some of the chief causes of forgetting.

Many cases of forgetting are in actual fact due, not to disturbances in the memory process itself, but to inadequate learning. It is, of course, rather obvious that, other things being equal, ease of recall will vary with the degree to which the material has been originally learned. If we particularly want to remember a telephone number, for example, we will repeat it to ourselves until it 'impresses itself' on our memory. Most of us could still rattle off multiplication tables, poems, and other relics of our early schooldays simply because this material was drummed into us by repeated learning. Repetition in fact leads to *over-learning* which facilitates later recall. This is merely another way of stating the truism that we will never remember what we have not learned sufficiently in the first place. At times we may find ourselves unable to recall an event simply because it has never been consciously registered in the first place. Habitual actions, such as winding one's watch, switching off lights before going to bed, locking the car door and so on are so repetitive and practised that the action may be insufficiently registered.

Although we have already said that long-term memories are more permanent and durable, there is some suggestion that the loss of some well-established memories may occur as a result of destruction or *decay* of the specific structural memory traces in the brain. Such isolated islands of forgetting would be associated either with the general deterioration of the nervous system with age, or as a result of cerebral damage due to injury or disease of the brain. Inability to recall an event does not of course necessarily imply that the memory trace has been destroyed. Some memories may be still well retained but temporarily inaccessible. This happens frequently in cases of concussion where the loss of specific memories is temporary. A similar short-lasting effect sometimes follows acute emotional shock, and a more self-directed form of selective forgetting due to emotional conflict has already been discussed under repression.

Perhaps one of the principal causes of forgetting is that caused by *interference* with the memory trace. We have already commented upon the vulnerability of information during the short-term phase of memory to interference by the arrival of fresh information. The effect of interference of new learning on previously registered data can continue for some time, particularly if both sets of data are rather alike. The term *retroactive inhibition* is used to describe the the influence of new matterial on previously learned material which has not had time to consolidate. For example, if we were learning some material in anatomy and followed it by learning some material in physiology, we would then expect retroactive inhibition to be high, as the similarity between these two subjects would tend to cause confusion. If the learning of anatomy were followed by learning in, say, psychology there would still be interference in the memory process, but not to the same extent, due to the lack of similarity between these two subjects. The most favourable conditions of remembering would occur if no activity at all followed the learning of the anatomy material until it had a chance to become consolidated. This reasoning leads to the suggestion, popular with students, that learning periods should be broken up by rest periods. If we do not plan our learning to exclude as far as possible the interference of related material then some distortion in recall will operate. The schoolboy who attempts to memorize names of historical figures first and then turns his attention to the name of geographical locations, may find himself writing in his next day's examination paper that Gandhi is a river in China.

In the foregoing discussion we have perhaps tended to view memory as a relatively mechanical operation, divorced from the remainder of the individual's personality. Although this approach is useful and effective in stimulating studies of the manner in which individuals process and store information, it is as well to remind ourselves that memory is a dynamic process, partly dependent upon the individual's attitude of mind. We may have to study for an examination material for which we have no use other than to answer the examiner's questions. Such a situation, of course, implies that there is something wrong in the syllabus or in our interpretation of it. In such circumstances we may be compelled to learn the material well enough to allow us to recall it accurately during the examination. If, however, it is of no further relevance we are more likely to forget it a short time after the examination is over. The lack of personal interest in the subject and its apparent irrelevance to our future lives produces a state of temporary retention only. Looking back on my own schooldays I can think of many subjects which were painstakingly 'swotted up' at the time for examination purposes. This was merely a waste of time and effort for, although my work achieved it short-term purpose, it did nothing to increase my permanent knowledge. Perhaps these memories are still stored somewhere in my brain but they are certainly inaccessible.

Many difficulties in remembering entail not so much forgetting as such but distortion of the original event. We commented earlier on the fallibility of perception which can lead people to observe the same situation quite differently. Memories are even less reliable than the original perception for the intervening time can play strange tricks on our memory. I am reminded of an aspect of my own work which provides a weekly reminder of this unreliability. Each week we hold a case conference during which a particular case is presented for discussion. Each member of the staff present at the meeting is usually obliged to put forth his views on the case and the meeting ends in a general exchange of ideas. Everything said at these meetings is taken down verbatim by a secretary (at other meetings we have employed a tape recorder). It is a most instructive and chastening experience each week to compare one's memory of what one has said at the meeting with the true record as taken at the time of the meeting. The usual finding is that one has conveniently forgotten the views which were criticized and rejected by other senior staff members. One also finds the opposite effect where one has padded one's memory of the event to include very clear thinking and praiseworthy ideas which were never actually uttered. In other words, we actively select from the material committed to memory so as to make out memory of past events as pleasant and as self-satisfying as possible. The longer the time interval between the event and the recall the more we are liable to distort our remembering in this way. This brings us back to the influence of our feelings and attitudes on our memory which we have already discussed under repression. There is little doubt that a great deal of forgetting is caused by repression of unwanted memories which threaten our self-esteem. What we remember will depend in great measure upon what we wish to remember.

The fallibility of the memory process also throws light on the question of how far back in our lives we can remember. People argue with great conviction that they have retained memories of events which occurred when they were infants. In actual fact it would seem that the capacity to retain a memory image of past events does not develop until around the age of 2 years. We have seen earlier that, in the case of the very young child, there is no memory process at work at all. During the second year of life the child is gradually able to recognize objects and events which are repeated but it is only later that the child can actually recall events clearly in their absence. Even then the span of retention appears to be very limited and it takes some time before the child is able to remember anything over a longer space of time. Nevertheless people do have adult memories of events which did take place at early infancy and we might well ask how this is possible. The answer would seem to lie in the unreliability of the memory process over a long period of time. Let us say that something particularly interesting or amusing occurs when little Willy is 8 months old. The rest of the family take note of the event which is usually something of the order of Willy emptying his soup plate on auntie's new dress. Later, at the ripe old age of 3 years, the incident will be recollected and retold with relish by the family as evidence of little Willy's early promise. If the household is a normal one, and the incident embarrassing enough, it will probably be recounted in detail at various times to unsuspecting visitors. The 3-year-old Willy will remember these accounts of his deeds but, as the years pass, he will come to believe that the memory relates to the original incident. As an adult William will be in a position to continue the legend which is now cited as evidence of his amazing memory.

Another type of memory distortion is the experience known as *déjà vu*. This describes the vague feeling of familiarity which arises sometimes in a situation of which we have had no previous experience; the 'I have been here before' feeling which starts us thinking about reincarnation or seeing into the future. The most likely explanation of this experience is the much less exciting one that it is a memory disorder based upon faulty recognition. Let us say we are travelling in a car through unfamiliar territory. We pass through a street, by a particular house, and quite suddenly we feel that it has all happened before. The same can apply to something someone has said which gives us an uneasy feeling that we have lived through this situation before. Usually there are some similar features in the present situation which resemble a past situation previously experienced. The street and the house are associated in some respects with a past experience. Instead of recognizing this, and recalling the past situation with its differences as well as its similarity to the present one, we instead experience only a vague sense of unaccountable familiarity with the present situation. The fact that *déjà vu* experiences are most common when we are tired or emotionally disturbed helps to explain the failure to relate the two situations correctly. In more severe cases of emotional disturbance such disorders in recognition are particularly frequent.

Memory and Brain Damage

As memories are stored in the brain we might expect the forms of memory disturbance demonstrated by patients with known brain injury or disease to advance our understanding of the relationship between memory functions and cerebral structures. We have already noted that the diffuse brain damage which accompanies ageing tends to exert a fairly marked effect upon the efficiency of the short-term memory system. Most studies of the effects of more specific types of brain damage have substantiated the findings of Penfield (1954) that the integrity of the temporal lobes is vitally important for memory storage. Earlier investigations in this field established that memory defect was noticeable in patients with damage to both temporal lobes, unilateral damage having apparently little effect on retention. This finding has been greatly clarified by the findings of a number of later investigations which suggest that the two temporal lobes differ in their specialized roles they play in memory. Such studies have demonstrated that damage to the left temporal lobe tends to be associated with impairment in the retention of auditory, verbal material while right temporal damage leads to impairment in memory for visual material (Milner, 1958, 1960; Kimura, 1960, 1961). Such differences in the modality specialization of the two temporal lobes may explain why learning and memory is often surprisingly little affected by extensive damage to one temporal lobe. Presumably subsequent learning is mediated mainly in the alternative sensory channel so that a falling off in visual memory is compensated by an increasing use of auditory memory via the intact temporal lobe. It is tempting to speculate that the noted prominence of poor visual memory in the elderly may be connected with right temporal lobe damage.

Aids to Learning and Remembering

I am often asked during lectures to give some hints towards improving one's learning capacity and one's ability to remember the material learned. Unfortunately there are no magic formulae we can produce to achieve such a purpose but we will close this chapter by mentioning a few points which might usefully be kept in mind as aids to efficient learning and remembering.

1. Concentration and Interest

As we have already said, we cannot hope to have a good memory of any material unless this material is first well learned. Many people say that this is, in fact, their chief problem in that they find it difficult to concentrate on the material in the first place. If a person is physically and mentally healthy, concentration is largely a matter of his present interests and his outlook for the future. This can be easily demonstrated by the fact that some students will sit through an hour's lecture and be unable to concentrate on it sufficiently to remember any part of it an hour later. At the same time they will sit through a three-hour cinema programme in the evening and weeks later be able to give a very good account of the films. Some members of the fair sex may be unable to give an account of a conversation a few days after it has occurred but they will be able to give a minute description of the clothes worn by the other person. In other words, if we are interested in the material to be learned or if it fits in with out future aims and goals, concentration will follow naturally.

We might object that much of the material which one has to learn is not interesting and, therefore, it is difficult to work up an interest which will allow one to concentrate. The material itself need not be interesting as long as it has some meaning and significance to the individual in terms of his personal life. For instance, delinquent children of low intelligence find it almost impossible to learn arithmetic in school but, when the same lesson is given in the context of how to work out money made on betting on horses or how to work out permutations for football pools, the arithmetic is easily learned. The same might be said of the material learned by the nurse in that if she is able to relate the material learned in the classroom to her every-day life, to her work, to her relations with others in general, and to widen her understanding of herself, then the material will be learned and remembered to a greater extent.

2. Rote Learning

Unfortunately, we must admit that in the case of some material which we must learn it is virtually impossible to imagine it stirring up interest. This might be said to be true in the case of the person who is faced with the task of remembering or memorizing the bones in the human body, although it is possible to teach this material in a more meaningful and interesting way. Some material does, however, seem to demand what we call *rote learning*. By rote learning we mean over-learning to such a degree that the memory is mechanically fixed in our mind. This, as we have already said, is the way we learn the alphabet, multiplication tables, and even poetry at school, and some types of material may be more easily digested in this way.

3. The Importance of Insight

The use of rote learning is very limited as it involves memorizing without any insight into the meaning of the material. As opposed to this, true learning involves not only remembering the material but seeing it as a meaningful whole. It also means that the material which is learned is capable of being applied to other problems. For example, it might be possible by rote learning to memorize the gist of the chapter on adolescence and to do the same with the later discussion on social groups. If, however, we have learned our material in this meaningless way, we are completely stumped when faced with an examination question on the adolescent as a member of a social group. It is, of course, a primary responsibility of those who teach to ensure that learning is accompanied by insight. We have already referred to some of the means to this end in our comments on participation learning but we will elaborate these remarks in our next point.

4. Active v. Passive Learning

On the whole, learning will be more effective if it is active rather than passive. We may make our learning more active by reviewing our material at frequent intervals; that is, when we read a passage in our lecture notes or a book, our memory of this passage will be greatly strengthened if we take the bother to stop and summarize what we have just learned. Another way of making learning active is to discuss what one has learned with others. In this way our attention is drawn to different parts of the material which have been inadequately or incorrectly learned. It is also valuable to apply the material learned in practice. For example, our anatomy and physiology lectures will be more meaningful and will, therefore, be remembered better if we apply them to our own bodies or those of other people. Finally, one cannot over-stress the importance of writing notes and critical reviews of the material which we have learned. This forces us to order our thoughts and summarize our ideas in a few words and thus greatly aids our later remembering.

5. Incentive and Accomplishment

A great deal of what we have already said can be summarized by emphasizing the necessity of having a definite goal or incentive in mind when learning. In nursing the goal may be simply to be qualified and efficient or it may take the form of the longer term goal of keeping one ambitious eye on matron's cap. The nurse who drifts aimlessly into her training is likely to continue to drift in no set direction, merely squandering her energies upon wasteful and unenthusiastic learning. The knowledge of a goal is, however, not enough in itself. Most of us are human enough to need the further incentive and reassurance of seeing ourselves making steady progress towards our goal. This reassurance may take the form of examination marks, praise from our seniors, or a subjective awareness that we are becoming more efficient at our work.

6. Planned Learning

As recall is dependent upon learning it is imperative that our learning methods should be as effective as possible. Short planned learning sessions where we set ourselves the task of covering a specific amount of work are likely to be more rewarding than less frequent and more lengthy periods where we measure progress merely by the time we have spent slumped over our books. Our learning periods should also be methodically spaced so as to avoid the interference caused by retroactive inhibition. Finally, we should remember that mental fatigue is invariably an attitude of mind rather than a barrier which forcibly limits our attainments.

7. Memory Systems

Sometimes despairing students ask if there are no 'systems' which they could use to improve their memory. As a 'bad' memory in itself does not actually exist there is not likely to be any way of improving one's memory. Poor memory usually denotes either faulty learning or a lack of interest in the learned material. Often, of course, it also denotes bad teaching. 'Memory systems' do, however, exist according to advertisements in the daily press which promise to 'build up your memory for you'. Most of these systems are based upon some variation of mnemonic learning. Most of us have used mnemonic devices at some time to assist our memory. The idea behind them is simply to replace the material which is difficult to recall by symbols which are easy to recall. Our recollection of the symbols will then guide us to recall the material associated with them. As a child I learned the musical staff by the mnemonic system of remembering that the notes on the spaces spelt f-a-c-e and the notes on the lines were the first letters of the phrase 'Every good boy deserves favour'. I also learned the days of the months by memorizing the familiar jingle 'Thirty days hath September. . . .' This, of course, is rote learning and if I am asked today how many days are in May I have to go over my jingle from the beginning. In other words, it has never really *taught* me the number of days in the months. Another drawback of mnemonic systems is that they may sometimes defeat their own ends. At one time I used to have dealings with a lady named Mrs McInnes. For some reason I could never remember her name so I resorted to using a mnemonic device. I associated her name with Guinness, a word more near to my heart, in the belief that this would be remembered and allow me to recall her name. The device worked but in the wrong direction for, thereafter, I persisted in calling the the poor lady 'Mrs Stout'.

8. Examinations

Examinations are often rather trying experiences and we will close with mentioning three little hints which are often helpful in this situation. In some cases a person becomes anxious and emotional when faced with a set of examination questions. Although he has learned the material he finds himself suffering from a complete memory block where his mind seems empty. This is caused by anxiety and emotional panic but it may cause further anxiety and panic as the person struggles to revive his memories. The best procedure when faced with a memory block, then, is to endeavour to relax for a short time and to think of something entirely different to allow the anxiety to pass over and the memory to start ticking over again. Secondly, it is always a good idea to read through the examination paper until one finds a question which one thinks one can answer and immediately start on this ignoring the rest of the paper. By the time we have answered this question we are more relaxed, at ease, and more confident to face later more difficult questions. Finally, it is a useful idea to rote learn, or overlearn, definitions or any other small parts of our material which can be used as opening phrases of answers. This, again, allows us time to settle down and the writing out of, say, a definition arouses other associations connected with it in our mind and 'triggers off' our memory on that particular subject.

Concluding Remarks

Studies of the learning process produce some general rules which improve our understanding of the functions of learning and memory. We are, however, again faced with the fact that we cannot study any psychological process as if it were isolated from the rest of the individual personality. Learning is fundamentally dependent upon interests, aims, and attitudes and these are in turn a reflection of our general individual outlook. Learning is also an active process which involves not only the whole of the individual's personality but his relations with others in his environment. The aim of true education is to increase maturity by helping the individual to develop his capacities and to think for himself in an adult way. The function of the educator is not merely to transmit information and knowledge. His true function is to act as a mirror which will reflect his own experience and knowledge of life in such a way as to make students more critically appreciative of the range and scope of their own minds.

QUESTIONS

1. Discuss the distinction between the psychological and physiological limits in human performance. How would you apply this distinction to the question of fatigue arising within the nursing group?

2. To what extent might the personality of the ward sister or nursing tutor affect her efficiency in successfully instructing the trainee nurse?

3. Describe and compare active participation learning with passive didactic learning. Describe how the merits of participation learning can be put into practice in nursing training.

4. To what extent might the study of learning and remembering as outlined in this chapter assist you in dealing effectively with your nursing studies?

11. The Process of Thinking

One of the most important abilities which raises man above other animals is his highly developed capacity for thinking or reasoning. This capacity has allowed him to shape his environment to suit himself while other forms of life have had to adapt themselves directly to their environment. Thinking is the last mental process we will consider and it occupies its rightful place in the chain of mental activities we have been dealing with in this section. We do not merely perceive, learn, and recall material; we put it to use, transforming it into new forms by our thinking. Thinking is not, of course, an isolated mental function, being basically linked with other processes which we have already discussed. Thus we have already referred indirectly to thinking in our previous discussions on such subjects as learning, intelligence, motivation, etc. Here we will confine ourselves to mentioning a few aspects of thinking upon which we have not already touched.

Directed Thinking

Asked what they are thinking of, people sometimes reply 'My mind's a blank!' In actual fact it is doubtful if our mind is ever a blank for it is an almost impossible task to think about nothing. Indeed, the very phrasing of the idea of thinking about nothing in itself reminds us that we are always thinking about something. It is true, however, that a great deal of our day-to-day thinking takes the form of undirected thinking. When we describe ourselves as thinking of nothing we really mean that we are thinking of nothing in particular, letting our thoughts take their own direction without focusing them deliberately on any specific issue. Many of our daily activities are also carried out by habitual reactions which require no deliberate effort of thought.

Although we are constantly in a sense thinking we are not constantly *reasoning*. Reasoning occurs when some form of an obstacle blocks the way to a desired goal. The less obvious the solution to the problem the more will reasoning play a part in its solution. Reasoning is then a conscious and deliberate focusing of our thinking on a specific problem which requires to be solved. We have already alluded to the reasoning process in our previous discussions on learning and intelligence. From what we have said before we can conclude that reasoning depends upon the perception of the relevant data concerning the problem and the combining of the essential data in the correct way. If we are asked, for example, to explain the best procedure for nursing a patient with a specific illness we first gather together in our mind all the data we have learned which appertain to the condition in question, ignoring all other data which are irrelevant to the situation. We then arrange these data in a way which will be best adapted to the needs of the particular patient, taking into account such factors as the patient's age and general health. By this method we finally arrive, by a process of reasoning, at the most satisfactory solution to our problem.

It is perhaps worth repeating here that, in the case of reasoning, as with other mental processes already discussed, the central feature is one of *inhibition*. The information which will lead to the solution of any new problem is usually to be found externally, in the nature of the problem itself, and internally, in the form of stored-up memories of past learning. Our ability to reach the solution will depend upon our capacity to inhibit what is irrelevant in these two sources of information. This allows us to concentrate on organizing the relevant information in a way which will lead to the solution. If we are tired or out of sorts, it is noticeable that we find this process of inhibition more difficult and complain rightly that we cannot concentrate our thoughts on the matter in hand. An individual's reasoning powers thus depend on the two factors of *inhibition* and *organization*. The latter is essentially tied up with our intelligence and is thus more a function of our basic intellectual capacity, while the former probably is nearer to a reflection of our state of mind at the moment. We might conclude from this that improvements in our reasoning would be most likely brought about by us seeking to improve on methods of sifting out what is relevant and productive in respect of the task in hand. A heightening of our inhibitory processes might make us, not only more adept at reasoning, but more reasonable creatures, for a great deal of biased and distorted thinking is due to our tendency to obscure our concentration with immaterial emotionally determined data irrelevant to the situation. In other words, solution of problems, particularly when these involve interpersonal situations, reflect more what we want to think and find rather than an objective picture of fact. Our powers of inhibition, like our intellectual capacity, may of course be ultimately limited by our constitution and our biochemical make-up. The processes at work in some of the severe forms of mental illness, for instance, appear to result in a reduction in the inhibitory potential of the cerebral cortex. As one intelligent schizophrenic patient remarked to the author, 'I start off thinking about something, but I never get there. Instead, I wander off on the wrong direction and get caught up with all sorts of trivial things that may be connected loosely with what I started out on but have nothing to do with the line I want my thoughts to follow. When I am trying to think I am like a railway engine running on a line where someone keeps changing the points'. One could not ask for a more vivid description of failure in concentration than that contained in the last sentence.

The reasoning process may become ineffective in a number of ways but psychological investigations have shown that the greatest barrier to effective reasoning is the adoption of a wrong initial assumption to which the individual rigidly adheres. We have already seen that reasoning involves a great deal of trial and error thinking. After discarding the data which are irrelevant to the problem we next proceed to try out various combinations of the relevant data in our attempts to find the solution. Often our thinking goes wrong because we slavishly follow one particular combination which does not lead to the solution. If we give a young child a set of building blocks of different sizes he may attempt to build a column by placing the larger blocks on top of the smaller ones. Time after time the child will persist in this approach only to see his construction collapse. His rigid adherence to the wrong principle prevents him seeing the correct way to combine the blocks to form a stable structure. Very often we find our own mental construction collapsing about us for the same reason (or the same lack of reason) until, like the child, we turn away frustrated at our lack of success. Effective reasoning demands flexibility and open-mindedness in the approach to any problem. The successful thinker is often the person who is most adaptable and does not allow himself to be trapped in blind alleys of his own making. We are again led back to the fact that education must encourage the student to reason for himself and to approach each problem with a flexible, adaptable attitude. The psychologist, Wertheimer (1945), strongly criticized the type of school education which he thought discouraged the development of active thinking in children. He referred to the over-emphasis of rote learning and mechanical drill which 'induces habits of sheer mechanized action, blindness, tendencies to perform slavishly instead of thinking, instead of facing a problem freely' (Wertheimer, 1945). Educational methods have improved somewhat since, and to some extent because of Wertheimer's criticisms. This is particularly so with nursing education where training is now based on producing understanding and insight instead of merely blind learning of sets of rules and procedures. The nurse of today accepts and receives explanation of the reasons for nursing procedures where once there was a tendency for her to carry out actions 'just because you are told'. Perhaps, however, if a relative outsider may be allowed a faint criticism, present day nursing training still tends to produce more rigidity and inflexibility of thinking than need be. Several doctors have admitted to me their concern that the nurse in training is too often taught her medical knowledge in black and white terms. Opposing views exist in all sciences and certainly medicine is no exception. Many aspects of medical theory and practice vary from one authority to another and, in some cases, there is wide diversity of opinion. That such disagreement and lack of certainty should prevail is a healthy sign which is essential to the continual advance of medicine as a science. One can well understand the damage which might occur if the nurse were faced with conflicting views at every turn at the beginning of her training. The result would only be to destroy her confidence in medicine as an exact science, for she would have no way of knowing the necessity and ultimate value of disputed opinion. An equal danger, however, lies in the other direction. If too much stress is laid on making all aspects of the subject matter appear exact and clear-cut the over-simplification may lead to rigid, inflexible, and at times erroneous thinking on the part of the nurse. I meet the same situation in my own subject when I find that some psychology lectures given to nurses contain material which is so simplified as to be incorrect. The influence of heredity and environment on intelligence is a little complicated to explain but to avoid the difficulty simply by saying that one's I.Q. is inherited and decided at birth is to be understood only at the price of misleading the student. Such over-simplification is also an insult to the student in its implication that he lacks the capacity to grasp the full explanation. Apart from mis-educating the student over-simplification may eventually defeat its own object for, if the student later learns that what was once taught as fact is little more than fiction, confidence in the subject is likely to be greatly diminished. Naturally it would never do if the nurse had to consider the full pros and cons of every procedure before she carried it out. One can imagine the poor patient awaiting an injection while the nurse stood back contemplating its action, side effects, possible alternative treatments, and so on. It does no harm, however, to accept the fact that many of life's issues cannot be fitted into separate compartments labelled right or wrong. Flexibility of mind is an asset which is essential to the development of healthy thinking habits.

Creative Thinking

Human knowledge continually advances because some individuals are able to produce new ideas which allow man to step-off in a new direction in his attempts to understand both himself and his environment. It has been suggested that about one half of all unique contributions in science and the humanities are made by a relatively small group, representing no more than 10 per cent of those engaged in the occupation involved. A discussion of creative thinking follows well on the heels of our previous remarks on the importance of flexibility in thinking for thinking must step outside the bounds of established thought to become original and creative. Those who add to the world's stock of knowledge do so often by their non-acceptance of the false assumptions which have limited previous thinkers in their subject. Let me illustrate this with a rather ridiculous example which nevertheless makes the desired point. The following story is told to a group of people. 'The detective opened the door of the flat. At one glance he took in the situation. The two bodies lay on the divan, one dead and the other drawing a last despairing breath. The remains of a shattered glass container lay in pieces on the floor. A cat crouched on the window-ledge as if frozen by the sight of the disaster in the room. The detective knew it was deliberate murder, and he knew the identity of the killer.' Most people will regard the story as incomplete, saying that too few facts are presented to explain either the murder or the identity of the murderer. Some, however, will have no difficulty in seeing the 'trick' which has thrown the others off the scent. The story becomes meaningful and the solution clear when we realize that the two bodies were of goldfish whose bowl the cat has pushed over. The solution only appears difficult because we tend to adopt the wrong initial assumption that the victims were human. The story may be ridiculous but there is little doubt that a great deal of our thinking is limited by our original assumptions. The creative thinker is flexible enough to consider all aspects of a problem, accepting nothing at its face value without critical appraisal. So often our first response on hearing of someone else's original idea is 'Why didn't I think of that, it's so obvious!' In a sense every new contribution to human knowledge is obvious, for the data upon which original thinking is based are often there for all to see. The creative thinker's contribution to any problem is to see it in an entirely fresh way, rearranging the data in a new pattern. Original thinking, then, depends upon maintaining a flexible and open-minded attitude to each situation, refusing to take anything for granted merely because it is generally accepted by others.

This notion, that the essence of creative thinking lies in the ability to perceive unusual associations between apparently diverse elements of a problem, has been described vividly by many creative thinkers of the past. In describing the creative process in art André Breton speaks of '. . . a marvellous capacity to grasp two mutually distinct realities without going beyond the field of our experience, and to draw a spark from the juxtaposition'. An even more picturesque description is given by Poincaré's introspections on creative thinking in mathematics. 'Ideas rose in crowds . . . I felt them collide until pairs interlocked, so to speak, making a stable combination. . . . To create consists of making new combinations of associative elements which are useful. . . . The mathematical facts worthy of being studied are those which reveal to us unsuspected kinships between other facts well known but wrongly believed to be strangers to one another. Among chosen combinations the most fertile will often be those formed of elements drawn from domains far apart.'

Many studies have been carried out in attempts to identify any distinguishing characteristics of highly creative individuals. There is a measure of agreement that creative people tend to have high I.Q.'s on standard tests, although many individuals with high I.Q.'s are remarkably non-creative. Not surprisingly, highly creative persons are described as non-conformists, as being highly imaginative and intuitional in their thinking, self-assertive and confident in their own judgements. Some studies of highly creative children suggest that they are more likely to come from a family background where individual divergences in opinion and behaviour are tolerated and are respected and where the children are encouraged by parental example to resist social pressures to conform. Some investigators (*e.g.* Torrance, 1963) have emphasized the many social and educational pressures which are exerted upon the creative child to sacrifice originality and fit in with the rest of the group. Indeed, Torrance suggests that a rigid group-oriented educational system may cause many potentially creative children to surrender their own original and productive modes of thought, rather than face progressive alienation from their group. Other psychologists, such as Getzels and Jackson (1962) point out that most teachers prefer to teach bright low creative pupils than bright high creative pupils, in so far as the former are less demanding and easier to handle.

It is worth adding here that our standard tests of intelligence tend to place the creative child at a relative disadvantage. Most test problems have only one acceptable correct answer, that laid down in the test manual. The original child may produce unique solutions to such problems which are unacceptable and thus give a misleading low impression of his ability. Some years ago, I was testing a little pre-school girl on an I.Q. test. One problem required her to complete the drawing of a little stick man by adding eyes, nose, mouth, arms, hands and legs. She added all the necessary parts but omitted the legs. Knowing that this omission would lose her I.Q. points, I asked if she were finished. She looked at her drawing, declaring 'Oh the poor man has no legs,'—and promptly drew in a pair of crutches. A highly original and clever response but, in terms of the test requirements unfortunately incorrect.

One final characteristic of the creative adult which should be mentioned is the spontaneous and uninhibited joy with which he approaches each life experience. Some observers have described this quality of freshness and wonder as almost childlike in its unbridled enthusiasm and speculated that regression to more primitive childhood modes of experience and expression is typical of the creative person. Barron (1972) correctly contradicts this impression when he insists this is not so much regression as 'progression with courage'. As Barron aptly puts it, such people 'bring their childhood along instead of leaving it behind'.

Another frequently heard misconception regarding the creative innovative thinker is that one can be too clever and original for one's own good in so far as 'genius is akin to madness'. Although it is relatively simple to recall a number of highly creative individuals whose career has ended in madness, systematic surveys indicate, if anything, a lower incidence of psychiatric illness among such people. Nevertheless, interesting similarities between creative and psychotic individuals have been noted. Both show highly unusual associations in their thinking, report odd body sensations (such as ringing in the ears, peculiar odours), a high incidence of mystical experiences, restlessness and proneness to impulsive outbursts. Several genetic studies have indicated a high incidence of creative, innovative thinkers in the biological relatives of schizophrenic patients. In a recent study, Claridge (1977) was able to demonstrate significantly positive correlations between scores on creativity tests and those on a test measuring psychotic thinking within a population of college students. Another study (Dykes and McGhie, 1976) produced evidence suggesting that one factor behind the resemblances in the thinking of psychotic and creative individuals is that they both tend to maintain a wider attention than normal, excluding little as irrelevant. For some reason, the creative individual is able to perform a wider sampling of available environmental input without it exerting any detrimental effects upon his performance. The psychotic, in contrast, finds his concentration impaired by his tendency to attend to all events in his immediate environment. Another difference between these two types of individuals lies in the degree of control the individual exerts over his attentive processes. While the creative person is able to focus his attention narrowly in conditions where effective performance demands concentration on one event only, the psychotic shows considerably less voluntary control over his attention.

Such findings have led some to postulate a common genetic link between schizophrenia and creativity. What may be inherited is a tendency to attend widely and to think in novel, innovative ways. If the individual is fortunate enough to find a vocation and way of life in which his idiosyncratic thinking is welcomed, he may be accepted as an unusual but gifted person. On the other hand, if he is unable to find a socially acceptable way of harnessing his deviant approach to things, he may become progressively isolated and finally be labelled as psychotic.

Undirected (Autistic) Thinking

Most of the psychological studies of normal thinking have been confined to the process of reasoning or directed thinking which we have been considering. Normal thinking is, in fact, traditionally viewed as being directed towards reality and as following the rules of logic and reason. It has been recognized that the abnormal thinking of the mentally ill is not adapted to reality and does not follow the same logical pattern. Abnormal thinking is often described as being *autistic* to differentiate it from normal thinking. Autistic thinking may be defined as 'a type of thinking dominated by subjective trends, the material being unconnected in its essential features by objective standards, *e.g.*, day-dreams' (Warren's *Dictionary of Psychology*). The familiar description of the psychotic patient living 'in a world of his own' thus has some point, for his picture of the real world is distorted by his inner needs and fantasies. This definition of autistic thinking would almost apply to the egocentric thinking of the young child who has not yet learned to adapt his thinking to the world as it really is.

A little reflection, however, soon shows us that adult thinking is not always as objective and logical as we might like to suppose. The type of thinking which occurs in the dream state is far from being adapted to reality. Autistic thinking can, as we have seen, occur in normal experience under artificial experimentally produced conditions, but we can easily find further evidence of autistic trends in the everyday thinking of the normal adult. We have seen that the very way we perceive the outside world may be greatly influenced by inner subjective factors such as our attitudes. Prejudiced thinking, rationalization, and projection are but further illustrations of reality distortion in normal thinking. Emotional disturbance of any type appears to interfere with the logical pattern of our thinking and make it less attuned to objective reality. A great deal of our thinking is, in fact, not directed to coping with our environment in a deliberate rational fashion. We all have our day-dreams, our inner world of reality in which we triumph over all the obstacles which we have tripped over in real life. Sometimes the day-dreams are so much more satisfying than life that we withdraw our energies from tackling our problems directly, finding it easier to deal with them in our fantasies. If we relax our attention and cease to focus our thinking on any particular subject we are apt to find thoughts 'tumbling through our minds' in an apparently illogical undirected way. When we are over-tired or under stress our thoughts seem to run away from us in that they no longer pursue a specific direction. Each thought arouses a number of apparently unconnected associated thoughts, the effect being to send our thinking off in tangents rather than in a straight line. To reason out any problem we have to restrict the trend of our thinking to a set course, ignoring or inhibiting the irrelevant associations which arise during the process. In using the word 'course' in the last sentence I may, for example, have aroused associated ideas of golfing. This, and other possible associations, I inhibited to allow me to follow the relevant line of thought. Obviously, if we allowed our thinking to be too undirected we would seldom arrive at rational conclusions. Rather than speak of two different types of thinking, autistic and directed, we might more validly say that these terms denote two *aspects* of thinking. We might indeed view the thought process as a continuum with wholly autistic subjective thinking representing one extreme and wholly rational objective thinking the opposite extreme. The thinking of the chronic psychotic patient would represent the autistic extreme while that of the ideal scientist would represent the completely reality orientated extreme. Most of us would fall somewhere between these two poles in that our thinking is affected by both subjective and objective factors. In some cases autistic and reality directed thinking may interact in a profitable way. The artist, for example, may utilize autistic thinking in his work which does not need to conform to the same logical framework as, say, the work of the mathematician. If the artist wishes to make his work comprehensible to others he will, however, require to translate his subjective ideas into some sort of objective sequence. While autistic thinking is essential to the production of art, and to spiritual experience in general, we must free ourselves from its influence if our thinking is to conform to objective standards. It is surprising how much adult thinking is dominated by autistic elements in the form of superstitions, prejudices, and other types of bias. Let us take a few examples of the lack of logic involved behind a great deal of human behaviour. Thousands of pounds a year are paid by the public to racing tipsters, fortune tellers, and others who, if their claims were genuine, would have no need to depend upon a gullible public for their living. Most superstitions are founded upon fact which had some rational basis in the past. The superstition of avoiding the third light from a match arose during trench warfare in the first world war when a match lit for any length of time invited a sniper's bullet. More than fifty years later people continue to refuse the third light from a match although the original circumstances no longer apply. Patent medicines have been sold which promise not only to mend a bewildering variety of physical ills but to 'cure' also such personality traits as shyness. The effectiveness of the claims made by advertising campaigns are a testimony to man's failure to temper his enthusiasms with logic. The widespread acceptance of the type of racial and political stereotypes mentioned earlier further illustrates the lack of realism in human thinking. An otherwise well informed and sensible adult, president of a large welfare club, expressed his belief to me that all mental illness was a result of 'bad living and venereal disease'. Few of the mental patients he was condemning hold views as irrational as the one he expressed. The nurse meets many completely illogical beliefs about illness and treatment which patients cling to with the utmost tenacity in the face of all logical argument. I can remember one man telling me that his doctor must be wrong in diagnosing rheumatism in his case for he had always carried a potato in his hip pocket.

The strength of such illogical beliefs is evident in their widespread existence. Under the rational shell of most adults there still lingers the egocentric echoes of the magical thinking of childhood. I must admit to an uncomfortable feeling as I walk under a ladder with a simulated air of calculated defiance of the fates.

In any profession such as nursing which demands accuracy, logical thinking, and freedom from subjective bias, it is imperative that our thinking should be as free as possible from such autistic sources of error. The nurse has a responsibility to her patients and to herself to direct her thinking along rational and controlled lines. The first step to controlling and directing our thinking is to be aware of the existence of non-rational forces and to recognize the influence these may have on our behaviour.

Thinking and Speech

Although the thinking process may be studied in a non-verbal setting by using sorting tests or other tests of concept formation, a great deal of our understanding of how a person thinks is arrived at by studying his verbal reasoning. Even if we are thinking silently, our internalized thoughts are constructed in the form of words. Our speech is the clearest and most direct expression of our thoughts, and certainly the simplest way of understanding how a person thinks and what he thinks about is to listen to what he says. It is of course true that a great proportion of our everyday adult speech appears to require little or no thinking. Earlier in childhood the relationship between speech and thinking is a great deal clearer in that the child can be observed in the process of learning to translate his thoughts into speech, so that they may be communicated to others. Gradually, however, the normal child learns to master the techniques of speech and to become sufficiently acquainted with language to be able to express himself easily and spontaneously without undue attention to the process of recoding thoughts into word sounds. Speaking becomes a habit and, like all habits, it is a process which can be carried on without much conscious attention. The habitual side of speaking is further helped by the fact that our everyday speech contains a great many conventional phrases and sequences of words which literally roll off our tongues without premeditation. If, however, we are trying to express ourselves on something new which does not merely involve the repetition of familiar clichés, the study of a person's speech utterances may tell us a great deal about his thinking. It is of course obvious that *what* a person says—the *content* of his speech—will give us some insight into what he thinks about. Recently, however, psychologists have become interested in the *way* in which a person thinks—the *form* of his speech. Again it is not possible for us to consider the significance of such studies in detail and many of them are extremely technical, involving complicated linguistic analyses. We might, however, refer briefly to the work of Goldman-Eissler (1956, 1958, 1961) who has approached the study of speech habits in a rather unusual and interesting way. Goldman-Eissler became interested in what one might call the flow of speech or the personal rhythm of the individual speaker. In order to study this in a more systematic way, she utilized a technique which allowed the rhythm of a person's speech to be translated on to a visual record. In examining such visual speech records, Goldman-Eissler noticed that normal spontaneous speech was discontinuous in nature in that our speech is broken up by pauses of different durations. Some of these pauses are dictated by our breathing and others by the grammatical structure of language which causes us to pause, for example, at the end of a sentence. Many of the hesitations in speech were not, however, of this nature and indicated that speech normally consists of short groups of words interspersed with pauses which have no apparent connection with the grammatical structure of language. Indeed, Goldman-Eissler's studies suggest that almost half our speech takes the form of phrases of less than four words, while three-quarters of our speech is in phrases of six words. She concluded that such pauses in spontaneous speech must be meaningful and as much a part of the communication process as the speech utterances themselves. If such speech pauses were an integral part of the speech process, it seemed likely that one of their functions might be the planning of speech and that a study of the distribution and significance of such pauses would afford us some insight into the process of thinking itself. In a series of further experiments, Goldman-Eissler has been able to show that the words following a speech pause were usually at a higher level of abstraction and conveyed more information to the listener than the words occurring before a speech pause. The pauses then indicate the points in a person's speech when he is actively thinking. We often associate hesitations in speech with difficulty of expression. The person who speaks fluently with very little hesitation may often be regarded as being more intelligent and more likely to convey original and useful ideas in his speech. Goldman-Eissler's studies indicate that lack of hesitation of speech may indicate a low level of thinking or merely longwindedness. Hesitancy in speech tends to be associated with the attempt to formulate thinking in a concise manner, so that what is expressed contains a higher level of information.

Concluding Remarks

From our necessarily brief summary in this chapter we might conclude that human thinking is not always the rational deductive process it is assumed to be. Indeed, the more we study normal adult thinking in action the more we are impressed that it differs from abnormal pathological thinking only by degree. As soon as we are placed in a situation where we voluntarily or involuntarily relinquish all the normal control and direction which we give to our thinking, our thoughts follow the same subjective and often bizarre pattern characteristic of the thinking of mental patients. Our capacity to think clearly and thereby to deal effectively with our environment is influenced by our feelings, emotions, and the remnants of the prelogical type of thinking of childhood. Thinking which is directed to the solving of a specific problem in an objective rational way is denoted by the term 'reasoning'. Although our reasoning ability is obviously related to our intellectual level, it would, nevertheless, appear that most of us are limited in our thinking not by our intelligence but by our inability to retain a flexible approach to the problems which face us. Rigidity, blind mechanical learning, adherence to false assumptions, and automatic conformity to the views of others, are all factors which prevent us developing our thinking to its maximum level of efficiency. Possibly the single factor which most restricts us in our thinking is, however, that of a lack of confidence in our own views. So often it is not that we cannot think straight but rather that we are afraid to do so.

QUESTIONS

1. Comment on the importance of *flexibility* in effective thinking.

2. How would you distinguish between directed (rational) thinking and undirected (autistic) thinking?

3. Discuss some of the ways in which autistic elements limit our ability to think in a reasonable and adult manner.

4. Consider the significance of speech pauses.

Part Four
Social Groups

We have already emphasized in previous discussions the fact that all human beings are dependent on others from birth until death. This dependence is not only of a physical or economic nature, for it is also true that none of us can develop our personality without the presence of others. We do not work and play only to keep ourselves alive but also to obtain the acceptance, love, and affection of other people. In Chapter 1 we discussed the impact of the family group upon the child's development. However, as adults, we are at one and the same time members of a complex system of different groups. Such groups include social and recreational groups, political groups, religious groups, occupational groups, national groups, and so on. Our whole life tends to be influenced by the groups to which we belong. Man is, in other words, a social being and therefore the way in which he relates himself to others is of primary importance in obtaining an understanding of his behaviour. We cannot hope to understand individual behaviour unless we understand a little of the ways in which group membership affects the individual's life. In this last section of the book we will examine some aspects of the structure and function of social groups. The following chapter will deal in general terms with the interrelations between different groups and the internal relations between group members. The final chapter will take up the question of group morale and leadership.

12. Group Processes

Group Differences

Throughout our previous discussion we have continually emphasized individual differences which make each of us a unique individual whose personality and behaviour contain distinct features setting us apart from all others. There are, however, general patterns of behaviour which individuals have in common by virtue of their belonging to a specific culture or social setting. Some sociologists and anthropologists have suggested that these *culture patterns* have more effect on personality development than all other inherited or environmental influences.

One of the basic essentials for individual mental health is that we are able to adjust ourselves to the values and customs of the society to which we belong. As we develop we find it necessary to conform to the existing pattern of social conventions if we are to be accepted by others. We learn, in fact, a social code of 'do's' and don'ts' which guides our behaviour. On such social conventions we base not only our moral standards but our assessments of normal and abnormal behaviour. We tend also to assume that the conventional standards of behaviour in our own society apply to other societies.

It is true to say, as we did earlier, that our basic moral and ethical outlook is developed in childhood through the influence of the family group but the values of our parents often merely reflect the values of society as a whole. We thus grow up assuming that the norms governing our behaviour are absolute and universal, whereas many of them are in fact relative to the social and culture pattern in which we develop. It is important for us to remember that what is abnormal to us may be deemed normal by members of other societies. Homosexuality, for example, is considered by us to be an abhorrent and highly abnormal form of sexual behaviour while in some other cultures it is accepted and actively encouraged.

Most of the main social rules and taboos operating in any society have the useful and necessary function of encouraging forms of behaviour which hold society together while discouraging behaviour which would have the opposite effect. Such social sanctions then exert a healthy influence in helping us to live together in a socialized and harmonious fashion. There are, however, other social conventions which have less harmonious effects. I refer here to the multitude of minor customs which have a stifling effect upon individual expression. Often we are told that certain harmless actions are 'just not done' as if some irrevocable law had ordained it to be so.

The abnormal person is usually thought to be so because of his inability to adjust himself to his environment. As our environment consists largely of the social customs and conventions of the society in which we live, deviation from these community standards becomes the criterion of abnormality. Normal behaviour is then equated with conventional behaviour and to be 'different' may be regarded as equivalent to being abnormal. This criterion may work well in assessing many forms of abnormal behaviour; the extremely anti-social person is often abnormal in both a social and psychiatric sense. Many other perfectly healthy individuals do, however, find it difficult to conform to all the complex conventions of their society. They may be tolerated and accepted by others but at the same time be regarded as eccentric. A patient telling me about his work in a factory continually referred to one of his workmates as 'the queer fellow'. When I queried this the patient explained that this man was referred to in these terms throughout the factory. Asked if he knew the basis for the description the patient replied: 'They say he writes poetry.' If conventionality becomes the sole criterion of normality we tend to become intolerant and even afraid of the unconventional. Behaviour which is different from our own is regarded with suspicion and mistrust. What we do not understand we fear and ridicule. A short time ago, while lecturing to a class of young nurses, I noticed that one of the girls tended to be victimized by the rest of the class. She was the butt of the class's humour and the unhappy victim of numerous rather cruel practical jokes. This girl had committed two grave breaches of conventional behaviour; she stayed behind in the classroom each day to study any subject which she had not grasped and she did not go out with boys. These two deviations from the group behaviour were enough to prevent her being accepted by her fellow students. Over adherence to social conformity may ultimately restrict the scope for self initiative, independence of judgement, and mature development.

If we accept that such qualities are an integral part of psychological health, we arrive at the paradoxical position that what we often call 'normality' may be unhealthy.

This paradox is very evident to some psychologists who would seek to replace the adjustive concept of normality with what we might term an 'ideal' criterion of normal mental health. Under this rubric would be subsumed all the qualities which are associated with a healthy productive life in which the individual is able to 'actualize' himself as a developing person. As such self-actualization may include rejection of some conventional modes of behaviour, the ideally normal person may be radically different from our picture of the well adjusted normal person. Several studies of extremely well adjusted young people (Silber *et al.*, 1961; Grinker, 1962; Coelho, 1963) raise this point in observing that the very normal (in terms of social adjustment) students appear to be distressingly 'benign and over-accommodated' (Lazarus, 1969). Indeed, some such well adjusted paragons of the moral and social virtues appear to lack in their personal make-up the very character traits which are associated with highly creative people.

This latter point has been stressed by psychologists such as Frank Barron in his extensive studies of creative individuals. In his book *Creativity and Psychological Health*, Barron (1963) comments that '. . . rebellion-resistance to acculturation refusal to "adjust," adamant insistence on the importance of the self and of individuality is very often the mark of a healthy character. If the rules deprive you of part of yourself, then it is better to be unruly'. Later in the same book Barron reiterates the differences between the psychologically 'sound' and creative person (ideally normal), and the statistically normal (average) person. 'They (ideally normal people) are both more primitive and more cultured, more destructive and more constructive, occasionally crazier and yet adamantly saner, than the average person. . . . (They) are beset, like all other persons, by fears, unrealizable desires, self-conscious hates, and tension difficult to resolve. They are SOUND largely because they bear with their anxieties, hew to a stable course, and maintain some sense of the ultimate worthwhileness of their lives,' (Barron 1963).

We have already referred to the fact that social standards

of behaviour vary greatly between different societies. Members of other societies tend, therefore, to be regarded as highly unconventional when viewed according to our standards of normality. Mistrust of foreigners is, in fact, often based upon the same fear of anything which does not conform to our own ideas of normality. Although differences in language and ways of thinking are obstacles in the way of international understanding and tolerance, it is often the multitude of culturally determined characteristics which separates man from his fellows. The Frenchman is a 'queer fellow,' not because of his language nor his different form of government, but because he drives on the wrong side of the road and finds life dull without a mistress. The Englishman's worship of cricket and his preoccupation with weather forecasts are beyond the comprehension of other nationalities. While it is difficult to accept that our own beliefs and way of life are socially conditioned and not a part of the natural order of things, the recognition of the diversity of norms which guide human conduct allows us to be more tolerant and understanding of others. It also teaches us as individuals that we need not feel self-conscious or ashamed of our own way of life simply because it does not follow the pattern set by the majority.

The need for individuality, for self expression, and the right to 'do your own thing' is a strong motive force in today's society, particularly among its younger members. It is of course only two easy to criticize the conventional and decry the stultifying effects of over-conformity upon individual development. However, it is equally self evident that complete individual self expression is a myth and that the survival of society requires some degree of group conformity to social norms. It would seem that a healthy society is one which is able to make that difficult and always precarious balance between the needs of its members as individuals and as harmonious groups.

In the last chapter of the present volume we shall explore in more detail the whole topic of conformity and consider some of the more alarming effects of group pressures upon individual behaviour.

Group Loyalties

The social values and standards which guide our behaviour reach us through the agency of not one uniform group called society but through a variety of smaller groups of which we are members. Our differing social, occupational, political, religious, and other interests result in most adults being members of a number of groups each demanding some sort of allegiance. We are therefore expected to be loyal to the principles of our family, our church, our profession, our political party, and so on. As the standards of behaviour expected from us by each group may differ widely it is inevitable that group membership may involve the individual in some degree of conflicting loyalty. The principles of our profession may, for example, charge us to behave in certain ways which run contrary to the principles of our religion. At other times it may be difficult to reconcile our political standards with adherence to the conduct expected of us as members of a national group. The conflict is intensified when the conduct demanded by us as members of a group is at variance with our personal standards of behaviour. Group values and individual values may at times come into direct opposition. The pacifist in war-time finds that he can only remain loyal to his country's cause by surrendering his own personal beliefs. In a welter of group loyalties it is often difficult to remember that we also owe an allegiance to our personal integrity. Numerous occasions naturally arise where we must sacrifice our own personal desires to those of the larger group to which we belong. This is particularly true in relation to our work where our personal needs and ambitions may have to be held in check for the good of the group as a whole. We learn, in fact, that we can work more efficiently as a team than as a number of separate individuals pursuing our own ends. We also learn to accept and be guided by the authority of the group even when its commands run contrary to our own inclinations. An army can only function efficiently if private interests are submerged in the common interest. The same rule applies to any organized group activity from the running of a factory to the administration of a hospital. The rules and regulations which govern the behaviour of group members are passed down through the hierarchy of delegated authority which exists in any complex organization. Although in a hospital the rules which govern the work of the superintendent may differ greatly from those which the nurse learns to obey, they have the same basic aim of maximizing the total efficiency of the group's contribution.

It remains true, however, that in important issues individual loyalty to one's self is more important than group loyalty. Although we must continually make compromises between our own desires and the responsibilities which group membership incurs, such compromise has a limit. This limit is reached when our conduct as a loyal group member would lead us to transgress our own principles. A well co-ordinated and stable group allows its members the right to express their individual views even when they run contrary to those of the group. Thus, although our political system demands that members of parliament support the actions of their own party, this demand is elastic enough to allow any individual to oppose party conduct which they cannot reconcile with their own beliefs. This right of individual expression is the strength of democratic government and its absence the weakness of a totalitarian society which demands the absolute obedience of its members. Sometimes it is not easy to stand by one's own principles if it means incurring the antagonism of the group. The young nurse mentioned earlier had rather a bad time of it until her fellow students grew to respect her attitude to her work and her other divergent views. The reward of being true to one's self in this way is the intangible one of retaining one's self respect and personal integrity.

It is also tempting at times to shelve one's responsibility by denying it in favour of the group. The Nazi war criminals who put into action the orders of their superiors argued that they could not be held responsible for their behaviour. A young delinquent boy I once interviewed excused his part in a particularly brutal attack on two girls by saying that the gang to which he belonged would have turned on him had he not participated. In the final analysis we must accept the responsibility for our own actions. Some of the circumstances which may lead us to unwittingly surrender our self-responsibility will be considered in the last chapter.

Communication

We have already seen that group membership has a decided influence on our personality development. We adapt ourselves to the group's way of thinking which in time becomes the basis for our own actions. The shared interest in the group gives the members a common language and allows an easy interchange of ideas. This very process which encourages group solidarity tends, however, to create artificial barriers between members who belong to different groups with their own internal organization. Communication between groups is made difficult by the fact that each group has its characteristic modes of behaviour which may be quite different to those of other groups with which it comes into contact. We referred earlier to the misconceptions which arise when we as adults try to communicate with children. This barrier to adequate communication is caused by our tendency to assume that the child's thinking and behaviour are governed by the same logical rules which normally operate in adult thinking. The same situation, however, develops in communication between adults where the barriers are imposed by the basic differences in outlook of the various adult groups. The existence of different social classes in our society is nowadays maintained, not so much by differences in income or in educational opportunity, but by differences in interests, manner of expression, and standards of conduct. These differences arise to a large extent from the group ties we establish, making it difficult for a member of one social group to communicate with or understand the totally different point of view of members of another social group. Kinsey (1948) has illustrated the well-meaning damage which may occur when members of one social group try to impose their standards of behaviour on other groups. Often we tend to base our judgements as to what constitutes 'normal' behaviour on the too narrow and specific standards which operate in the groups to which we belong.

Even in cases where a number of groups strive after the same ideals their different traditional ways of thinking and behaving often preclude the clear form of communication which is necessary to ultimate understanding and agreement. If we are optimistic enough to believe that every nation in the world desires peace rather than face the total annihilation of another world war, we are still faced with the apparent inability of the national groups most concerned to understand each other's point of view. The western powers believe that democracy must in the long run prevail not only in their own sphere but throughout the world, while the eastern powers believe that communism must some day be accepted by all nations. The west is Christian in its faith while the communist bloc is mainly atheistic. Our conception of the state existing to serve the individual is largely opposed by communism's dictum that the individual is subordinate to the state. The west's description of itself as 'The Free World' is in opposition to the communist countries' belief that we are slaves of cruel capitalist masters. These are but a few of the major barriers to mutual understanding built on top of an accumulation of traditional differences in custom, habits, and conventional standards of behaviour, which combine to make international communication such a tremendous problem. The erection of such barriers to communication is a mutual construction and they can only be demolished by an effort on the part of both groups to step outside the now too narrow confines of their own standards to arrive at a consensus of opinion.

To illustrate the difficulties of communication between different groups we need not look as far as the international situation for we can find a more concrete and familiar example of communication breakdown in the organization of any hospital. We described a hospital earlier as consisting of a network of different groups each working in unison towards the common aim. Not only do we have the medical, nursing, administrative, domestic, and patient groups, but we have also a complicated hierarchical system of seniority with each staff group. Each of these groups is separated by fundamental differences in training, tradition, and occupational roles and these differences may also exist within the sub-groups. Any complex organization depends upon the existence of adequate channels of communication which will allow information to be effectively relayed throughout the different sections or groups. The army at war depends upon maintaining its lines of communication open at all times and the morale of its troops, the effectiveness of its activities, and the success of the whole campaign may depend upon an adequate flow of information. There is an oft-quoted story concerning the time-and-motion studies carried out some years ago to improve the effectiveness of the modern army. One of the investigators was given the job of studying the anti-aircraft batteries and he immediately noticed something which struck him as strange. Each man in a battery had a specific part to play in the battery's activities, with the exception of one man, known officially as No. 6, who appeared to have no clearly defined role to play in the team. After some research the investigator found the solution to No. 6's presence. In the days before these batteries were fully mechanized, No. 6's job was to take charge of the officer's horse. Now, years later, No. 6 still filled a place in the team, although the horse had long since disappeared. The story may not be authentic, but it illustrates the surprising results which may accrue from the inevitable side-tracking of communications which arise in any complex organization. This is no less true of the hospital and we will close this chapter with a brief consideration of some of the causes and consequences of communication breakdown in the hospital network.

The chief sufferer from inadequate communication in hospital is the patient and often it is the patient group which feels most isolated and bewildered by their ignorance as to what is going on, or by erroneous information. Obviously there must, for his own good, be some restriction on the information given to a patient coming into hospital. Nevertheless, a hospital is a rather strange and frightening place to most patients and relevant information, correctly given, may do much to dissipate the patient's exaggerated fears. Such information may deal merely with the organization of the hospital and seek to instruct the patient as to the meaning of some of the bewildering activities which are going on around him. Explanation may often seem time consuming and unnecessary, but it is surprising what misunderstandings can arise if we assume too much knowledge on the part of the patient. One old lady told me that she had spent several weeks in a hospital ward awaiting an operation. Each patient in the ward was transferred to another post-operative ward immediately after operation so they left their ward permanently when they were wheeled away to the operating theatre. The old lady, who had not been in hospital before, put the worst construction on what she saw and presumed that the patients did not return because they had died in the theatre. This so alarmed her that, when her operation was due, she refused to co-operate and would not believe the reassurances of the staff that her belief was illfounded. She was only finally pacified when taken to the other ward to see her missing friends alive and well on the road to recovery. Many hospitals now present new patients with a booklet detailing the hospital facilities and explaining, as far as possible, the system of treatments. A short conversation with a knowledgeable and understanding nurse is probably more effective in preventing any misunderstandings arising.

It may be profoundly more difficult to inform patients as to details of their own illness and the extent to which such information is given will, of course, depend upon the illness and the patient's capacity to accept and understand such explanation. Information can only be withheld successfully if there is adequate communication between the different staff members in contact with the patient. It is much more disturbing to patients if they are suddenly faced with unpleasant facts about their own condition through a remark let slip by a staff member who is unaware of the fact that such information has been withheld. A lack of staff co-ordination in communication may also result in the patient being given conflicting information from different staff members. There is, for example, nothing more aggravating and upsetting to patients to be told by the nurse that they are to be discharged from hospital in the near future, only to be given entirely different reports from sister and the doctor.

Communication difficulties can also be harmful to the patient if they are in a reverse direction. Patients tend to think of the hospital as a whole and to have little idea of the correct channels of information which exist. They may give a piece of valuable information to a staff member who may be a nurse, an orderly, or anyone else in contact with the patient. The patient then assumes that this information is automatically relayed to the hospital staff as a whole and be puzzled by the ignorance of the ward sister, doctor, or others who have no knowledge of the situation. If the recipient of the patient's confidence is unaware of its importance the information may go no farther and a piece of vital knowledge affecting the patient's condition may remain unknown. A more direct and often overlooked aspect of communication difficulty is seen in the patient's frequent inability to express his symptoms clearly. The question 'How do you feel?' is often extremely difficult to answer adequately and the patient's attempt to communicate subjective feelings may be highly misleading if taken at its objective value. An excellent example of what is entailed here is given in the following passage quoted from an American study of the dynamics of institutional life: 'One patient, upon becoming clear after a disturbed period, objected to the practice of physicians asking what bothered her. She said that she could not possibly tell because there were so many things and they were changing so fast. She then told an account of a friend who had been very severely injured with many broken bones and internal injuries in an automobile accident. In addition, her thumb was cut. In the hospital emergency room she was asked where she hurt and her answer was to hold up her thumb and say, "My thumb hurts". The patient who told this story said she understood this perfectly. When asked what is wrong, you have to answer something and you at least pick something definite' (Stanton and Schwartz, 1954). The trained nurse learns gradually how to assist patients in giving a true expression of their internal feelings.

When we come to discuss group morale in the next chapter it will be suggested that morale partly depends on each individual having a clear picture of the way in which their activities fit into the general pattern of group activity. Nurses sometimes complain that they 'feel out of it' as they do not have enough information as to their place in the total scheme of things. When this occurs it is usually an indication of a breakdown in the system of communication. The ward sister may be failing in her function of keeping her staff well informed as to the relevant facts regarding the patients or other general aspects of hospital routine and administration. The breakdown may occur at some other point in the line where, for example, the medical staff have neglected to ensure that the nursing group is kept adequately informed. Whatever the reason, lack of adequate communication results in the artificial isolation of some staff members and prevents them participating fully in the total pattern of activities. There is no doubt that some of these barriers to communication (particularly those which occur between the medical and nursing staffs) are traditional. Nurses complain that there is little point in the long reports on patients which they note down daily as the doctors either ignore them completely or give them only a cursory glance. The medical staff in turn are apt to deprecate the value of giving information to the nursing staff whom they say often seem uninterested and unenthusiastic. Often both these objections are valid and reflect unnecessary and avoidable wastage of time and energy. Nurses' reports, oral and written, are too often couched in stereotyped and meaningless terms due to the traditional formalities which surround the nurse-doctor relationship. The most valuable part of the nurse's observations may be omitted or disguised beyond recognition in traditional jargon and phraseology. This is partially true in mental nursing where the nurse's intimate and personal observations on the patients are of extreme value in treatment. Patients are reported in such meaningless traditional terms as 'impulsive' or 'hallucinating' which miss the whole wealth of information contained in the nurse's observations. If the nurse is helped to appreciate the importance of her own opinion of the patient's behaviour her reports soon become alive, free from conventional jargon, and describe not only the patient's behaviour but what lies behind it. The following extract from a mental nurse's report on the same patient at monthly intervals illustrates the changes that occur as the nurse gains confidence and learns to report her true observations. First report: 'Mary Bruce was impulsive towards the equipment.' Second report: 'Mary Bruce was standing in her corner banging a chair on the floor. She seems angry.' Third report: 'I don't think Mary bangs the chair on the floor because she's angry, but because she's frightened.' Later the nurses said: 'Mary always stays in the same place. When we go near her she looks fierce and bangs her chair on the floor. She's giving us a warning to keep away. She's very frightened of us for some reason and won't allow us within a circle of six feet round her. Now that we are not worried by her shouting and noise we go up to her and speak, and this seems to soothe her.'

This type of communication blocking is, however, a two-way process, the blame for which must be shared by the medical staff who sometimes either make little attempt to communicate with the nursing staff or, if they do, make their reports in an equally formal medical language which is often incomprehensible to the nurse. A great deal of this type of disruption in communication is nowadays being dissipated by the increased and more informal contact between the nursing and medical groups. Open discussion between the two groups, first during training and later during the day-to-day work in the ward, is allowing the maximum use to be made of the knowledge of each by a freer exchange of information and opinion.

A patient coming into hospital is forced to give up a great deal of personal privacy but retains the right to have personal facts relating to his illness treated in confidence. Because of this the doctor may feel that certain aspects of any case must not be passed on to other sections of the hospital staff. This imposes a certain amount of restriction on the free interchange of information which is reasonable and necessary if the patient's wishes are to be respected. The nurse may be denied access to such information and in most cases the secrecy does not affect the nurse's ability to carry out her duty towards the patient in an adequate manner. Sometimes, however, one feels that medical confidence may be over-respected. This point is again particularly important in mental nursing where details of the patient's private life may be highly relevant to his treatment. It has for long been a matter of grave concern to the medical authorities as to how much information it is necessary to give the nurse to allow her to appreciate the factors involved in her patient's condition. Some medical superintendents of mental hospitals deny the nurse any access to the patient's case history while others allow the ward sister to have free access and to use her discretion in communicating information to her nurses. One is inclined to feel that such concern is often needless and reflects the psychiatrist's unrealistic view of what goes on in the ward between patients and nurses. While attending a recent conference on mental nursing I heard a psychiatrist discuss with gravity the responsibility of the doctor to his patient's right for privacy. He declared that he would feel morally wrong if he were to divulge information to his nursing staff which a patient had told him in confidence. The perfect reply was put by a nurse who stood up to ask how much the nurse should tell the doctor of information confided to her by the patient. She went on to say: 'Many patients seem a little frightened of the doctor whom they only see now and then. They are with us all day and they soon start telling us all sorts of things about themselves which seem important in relation to their illness. However, they very often end up by saying: "Whatever you do don't tell the doctor that!" ' I have no doubt that the same situation arises in general nursing and that the nurse soon knows more of the patient's private affairs than any other member of the hospital staff.

The Dying Patient

Perhaps the most difficult of all communication problems is the question of informing the dying patient. Studies of the reaction of patients who are informed of the terminal nature of their illness indicate a great deal of individual variation. However, it has been commonly observed that reactions are often greatly shaped by the degree to which individuals see themselves as having realized their major life goals and commitments. In his book *The Meaning of Death*, Feifel (1959) concludes: 'The crisis is often not the fact of oncoming death per se, of man's unsurmountable finiteness, but rather the waste of limited years, the unassayed tasks, the locked opportunities, the talents withering in disuse, the avoidable evils which have been done.'

This may be part of the reason that elderly people often seem to be able to face their mortality with a great deal more sanguinity than younger people.

Many patients show an astonishing capacity to reject the reality of the situation when they are informed of the inevitable. They continue to entertain the firm conviction that the diagnosis is at fault, that a new treatment will suddenly appear, or any other phantasy which will, at least temporarily, block the pain of the reality. The protective value of the mechanism of denial should not be underestimated. It reduces the current stress level and may be the patient's way of indicating that he is not yet ready to deal with the situation. Denial may be a powerful stress reducer, not only to the dying patient, but to his relatives. In one study of the reactions of parents of children dying of leukaemia, it was observed that parents who completely denied the truth of the situation showed greatly lowered psychological and physiological signs of stress, as compared with other parents who accepted the inevitability of the outcome. However, the 'denial' parents showed a much more intense stress reaction when faced with the subsequent loss of their child.

An important point in this study concerns the increased stress put upon the 'accepting' parents by well-meaning relatives, friends, and some hospital staff. Either because of their own unwillingness to accept or simply to bolster the morale of the parents, these others would dispute the diagnosis, refer to miracle cures, insist the child looked better, and so on. This often put the unfortunate parents in the position of defending the reality of the diagnosis and its consequence and consequently feeling guilty that they appeared to be heartlessly condoning the death of their child.

As most nurses appreciate, there is no pat answer to the traditional question of how much patients should be told in this situation. One might argue that all patients should be fully informed to allow them both to develop their individual coping strategies and to deal effectively with what time is left to them. However, one must also accept the fact that not all of us can cope with the enormity of such knowledge and thereby respect the manner which the individual chooses to handle this crisis.

Professional training does little to qualify a nurse or doctor to deal effectively with this difficult situation, and many seek to avoid a frank confrontation with the patient on the issue of their probable death. In one survey, only 12 per cent of a large group of medical practitioners said that they would be likely to inform their patients of the diagnosis of a probable fatal cancer. In a somewhat paradoxical fashion, almost two-thirds of the same group of doctors stated they would wish to be fully informed if they themselves were in the patient's position. The majority of the 88 per cent of the doctors who stated that they would not inform the patient also said they would probably relieve themselves of the difficulty by informing a close relative, who could in turn choose how much to tell the patient.

Similar questions put to general hospital patients indicate that over 80 per cent say that they would wish to be fully informed by their doctor if their illness was found to be terminal. Of course, one might argue that many of these patients would feel differently if they were actually in the position of having a fatal illness. However, the findings of studies of terminal patients seem to deny this qualification.

Thus, in one U.S.A. survey (Gilbertson and Wangenstreen, 1961), about 80 per cent of fully informed terminal cancer patients said they were glad they had been informed. Knowledge of their true condition had allowed them to make necessary plans and to prepare themselves emotionally.

Although it would appear that many people are eventually able to adjust themselves to the anticipation of approaching death, it would be unrealistic to ignore that such eventual adjustment may be achieved only after a preliminary period of profound emotional distress. Part of this distress may be related only directly to the appreciation of the termination of life per se but more to the ways in which others may react to the situation. It is not uncommon for relatives and friends unwittingly to treat the dying patient as if he or she had already ceased to exist. In most cases the patient will feel less troubled if able to spend his remaining time with his family, particularly if the family are secure enough to continue to fully accept their ailing member as still a functioning member of the family. If home nursing is not possible, it is important that the dying patient is offered the same type of warmth, compassion, and interest in his relationships in hospital. The genuine and spontaneous interest of a nurse in the patient as a person may do more than tranquillizing drugs to comfort such patients.

The application of tranquillizers or anti-depressants in alleviating the distress of the dying patient may be a necessary and effective way of helping the patient over the acute phase of adjustment. However, if emotional distress is longer lasting, psychiatric intervention may be beneficial. Many psychiatrists who are experienced in dealing with other areas of human distress are able to employ their therapeutic skills to help the dying patient find sufficient inner resources to reduce his agitation or depression.

Finally, it is obvious that a strong religious faith may offer the greatest degree of comfort to the dying patient. Death may then be seen as a new beginning rather than the end of life. Even to many who are not bolstered by such faith, death may be viewed as a termination of life's stresses or simply as an unknown journey. One of the most succinct statements of this attitude is contained in a quotation from Socrates which closes John Hinton's (1967) interesting book on dying. At the end of his trial Socrates is being taken away, condemned to death. As he goes, he makes the following comment to his captors: 'Now it is time that we were going. I to die and you to live; but which of us has the happier prospect is unknown to anyone but God.'

Concluding Remarks

From birth onwards we are dependent upon others for our development. During infancy and childhood this dependency is a consequence of our inability to exist in a physiological sense without the support and care of adults. In adulthood our psychological development continues to be dependent upon our ability to make satisfactory relationships with others. This process of adjustment is brought about by a gradual adaptation to the communal standards of the group influences to which we are exposed. Being one of a group which shares the same outlook gives us the feeling of 'belonging' which is necessary for a stable and secure development. The very forces which unite us in groups do, however, tend to set artificial boundaries between us and our fellows who belong to different groups. These boundaries may be heightened by geographical distance so that we find it difficult to understand people belonging to other national groups whose way of life is different from our own. Even within our own society, however, there exist many similar obstacles to mutual understanding caused by our allegiance to differing social, political, religious, and occupational groups. Over-rigid adherence to group standards may result in us assuming that our own standards represent an absolute norm upon which we can judge the behaviour of others outside our group. Society can only function effectively if provision is made for a maximum flow of communication between the different groups of which it is composed.

QUESTIONS

1. Describe some of the ways in which our behaviour tends to be influenced by the social groups to which we belong.

2. Comment on any ways in which group membership might limit our tolerance and understanding of others.

3. Discuss the difficulties involved in maintaining effective communication within the structure of a hospital. Comment on the type of problem which tends to arise in hospital when adequate channels of communication are not available and suggest what steps might be taken to minimize such problems.

13. Group Morale and Leadership

Social groups vary greatly in their stability, some remaining united in the face of disruptive forces which lead to the disintegration of other groups. If we were asked to point to the one factor which decides the stability or instability of any group we should most likely refer to the level of morale which exists within the group. Group morale not only influences the internal cohesion of any group but also plays a large part in influencing the effectiveness with which the group carries out its activities. During the last war the countries involved devoted a great deal of energy towards maximizing the morale of their own armed forces while at the same time endeavouring by propaganda to minimize the morale of the enemy. During war-time psychologists carried out a great deal of research into this important question of factors contributing to group morale and we have since become more aware of the significant role that such factors play in civilian occupational groups. We shall devote the first half of this chapter to considering some of the main factors conducive to the maintenance of high morale in any group with particular attention to nursing morale. As a consideration of group morale leads inevitably to the role of the group leader, we will conclude with a short survey of the functions and attributes of leadership.

Factors Affecting Morale

1. Awareness of the Group's Objectives

A basic necessity for any group is a clear awareness of the objectives which the group is aiming to achieve. Most groups exist because they have a purpose which unites the individual members. It is then essential that each member is allowed to have a clear idea of what these purposes are. This was demonstrated in war-time where the most stable sections of our fighting forces were those (such as the Commando units) who were not only given clear-cut objectives to achieve but were able to appreciate the place of their actions in the total plan of war. Other war-time groups which were denied a clear sense of their own function showed a corresponding lack of stability and poor morale. In the complex organization demanded by modern warfare it is often difficult to prevent the feeling of isolation and bewilderment which arises from inadequate communication between different sub-groups. A common complaint among front line infantry sections during the last war was that the troops often had no idea of the contribution which their actions made to the total plan. In such circumstances co-ordination becomes increasingly difficult and the group becomes a series of unco-ordinated sub-groups with poor over-all morale. Modern industrial organizations face the same problem, for mass production methods involve small groups of people working together to produce a part, which is quite meaningless in itself, of the total product. Morale is greatly increased by enabling each sub-group to see the relevance of its work to the total scheme of production. This rule applies equally to the co-ordination of hospital activities. A hospital is made up of a vast network of sub-groups, each playing a vital part in the total aim of giving patients the best possible service. The main sub-groups (medical, nursing, and administrative staff) may have radically different roles to play, but their activities are interdependent and have a common aim. If the hospital community is inadequately co-ordinated the important links between the different staff groups break down, thus resulting in lower morale and a general falling off in efficiency. If, for example, the nursing group does not clearly see its place in the total therapeutic plan of the hospital, the morale of the nursing staff and eventually of the whole hospital, will suffer. Whereas, if the nursing group is given every opportunity of seeing its own activities in relation to the hospital system as a whole, there will be less danger of such feelings of isolation arising. What is true of the nursing group as a whole is also true of the many smaller groups of which the nursing group is comprised. Each ward and each department must be clearly aware of their place in the total pattern of activities. This question is, of course largely a matter of adequate channels of communication between the different sections of the hospital community. One of the most important of the communication links is that between the nurse's formal training and her work in the ward and we have already stressed the need for such co-ordination in an effective training scheme.

2. Awareness of One's Own Role in Relation to the Group

The previous point is equally true of individual members of any group whose morale will be higher if they can easily see the value of their own role in relation to the general function of the group. Thus the total group morale will be much higher if each member has a clearly defined part to play the group's activities. It is so easy for the reverse to happen as when, for instance, the young trainee nurse is allowed to feel that her own duties are of little importance. We already referred to this question in our earlier discussion on adolescence where we emphasized the need for constantly keeping the student nurse 'in the picture' by explaining the place of her work in the ward programme. Hospitals today take more care to provide an adequate 'feed-back' of information to nursing staff through the agency of staff discussion groups where medical, nursing, and administrative staff meet together to share their knowledge and iron out any misunderstandings which have arisen. Often one of the most valuable aspects of the ward sister's role is that she is able to relay back to her nurses information regarding patients and general hospital organization which she learns in her function as the ward representative. The necessity for individual participation in the group task is particularly evident in the setting of the mental hospital where the nurse's duties are less clearly defined in comparison with the general hospital. In a hospital in which I once worked the nursing morale in several wards was extremely low. The nursing staff felt that their work was not recognized and played a relatively unimportant part in the hospital's therapeutic activities. The situation was remedied by the arrival of a new member of the medical staff who raised morale immediately by attacking the sense of isolation responsible for the existing state of affairs. He organized a weekly meeting between his own medical staff and the nursing staff in his wards at which he gave a brief summary on each patient who had been admitted the previous week. The nurses were then asked to comment on their own impression of the patient and the meeting would end with the medical and nursing staff deciding *jointly* the best treatment to be given to each case. Not only did this interchange greatly raise the nurses' morale (and thereby the ward morale), but it ensured that the maximum amount of information was known regarding each patient before treatment was decided upon. As we have already remarked, it is often the most junior nurse who is in most intimate contact with the patient and who, therefore, can make a most valuable contribution to planning the most effective form of therapy.

3. A Sense of Progress

Individuals may unite in a group to reach a future objective but the group will not stay united unless the members are able to feel that they are progressing towards that objective. If the final aim of the group is a very long-term one morale will be strengthened by the periodic attainment of minor objectives which act as signposts of steady progress. The morale of our country during the last war was greatly enhanced by regular achievements which indicated that we were on the road to victory, although the end of the road was not in sight. Thus, a group may have a clear-cut objective to aim at which is, however, so remote that morale may fall and the group disintegrate long before the objective can be reached. The nurse's main objective is presumably to be efficient at her work and thereby to help her patients to recover. Before this goal can be reached she must cope with a long period of training which at times may seem to have no ending. Her morale is, however, kept up by the minor attainments which give pleasure in themselves and also signify that the final goal is nearer. Such attainments include successful progress in examinations, the praise and encouragement of her seniors, the gratitude of patients, and her growing confidence in her own efficiency. Even when her training is complete the now qualified nurse will probably set herself new objectives such as further promotion or some form of specialized training. Her objective may be more simply to see her patients benefit by her care. Whatever the nurse's aim she continues to depend upon an occasional sign of further progress to maintain her morale throughout her arduous duties. She may feel confident in herself that she is coping efficiently with her duties but a few words of encouragement from a senior nurse, a doctor, or from a patient may help her to feel that her efforts are appreciated and worth while. Very often those in charge of others forget that their job is not only to guide the nurse by criticism, however constructive it may be, but also to give praise where it is due.

The morale-boosting value of steady progress is again

perhaps particularly evident in mental nursing where the patients are often apt to be more chronic and where the static nature of their condition may offer little encouragement to the patience and skill of the nurse. One can visualize nothing more depressing than to be nursing patients in a chronic ward of a mental hospital whose condition remains unchanged year after year. In such a situation we would hardly expect nursing morale to be very high. Fortunately recent years have seen a tremendous change in outlook regarding the treatment of the chronic mental patient. Far from being 'the forgotten patients' the chronic patient is now receiving as much if not more attention than the short-term mental patient. The emphasis is now on keeping the chronic patient mentally and physically active during his stay in hospital and to provide as much personal stimulation as possible. The key figure in the rehabilitation of the chronic mental patient is the nurse who is now being placed in charge of small groups of patients. The new approach to chronic mental illness epitomized by the work of Bickford (1955) and many others has given the mental nurse a chance to maximize her contribution to the hospital's therapeutic programme and, as a result, the morale of the nursing group has soared.

4. The Effects of Adversity

Every group at some time or other comes up against obstacles and difficulties which impede its progress and test its stability. While such setbacks may weaken or destroy an already unstable group, the more stable group will respond with a strengthened morale and unity. Reverting again to the illustration of war-time Britain, we might remember that our war-time defeats, such as at Dunkirk, tended to make us a more unified nation and increased the national effort. Some years ago during as Asian 'flu epidemic, the hospital in which I worked was rather hard hit. Not only did the patients require more nursing but a large number of the nursing staff were themselves laid low by the epidemic. During these adverse circumstances the nursing morale was, paradoxically, at its highest. Nurses who were obviously unwell insisted on remaining to cope with heavier duties while those nurses in sickbay were demanding to be allowed back to their wards before they were fit to return. The temporary adversity had, in fact, unified the nurses and demonstrated the true stability of the nursing group.

5. Unity through a Common Hostility

Related to the previous point is the fact that group morale is often raised by the presence of a clearly defined enemy towards which hostility may be expressed. Not only does this allow the members to share a common feeling, but it also provides a convenient target for displaced feelings. Any tensions existing within the group can be relieved by the members displacing their aggression on to the common enemy. We have already cited Hitler's persecution of the Jews as an example of the morale-raising value of such a manoeuvre. In the hospital setting the common enemy is obviously disease. The destruction of an enemy is, however, a negative aim and it would appear that groups which are held together by mutual hate are less likely to survive than groups which have more positive and constructive goals.

6. Distinctive Symbols

Any factor which helps to differentiate the group from other groups tends to help in unifying the group and increasing morale. Most groups adopt some procedures which mark their members off from others. The gang of children which adopts a secret password and initiation procedure makes gang membership more exclusive in the same way as membership of adult groups (*e.g.*, Freemasons) often involves similar rituals. The symbols, rituals, and codes of conduct which surround many religious and political organizations have the same function. A distinctive form of dress also falls into the same category in that it gives the group members a common attribute which is not shared by outsiders. The traditional uniform of the nurse may not be everyone's idea of a fashionable form of dress but it does heighten the sense of group solidarity. The common training of all nurses and the ethical code which is a part of it probably serve a much more important function in increasing the cohesiveness of the nursing group. People, however, thrive on competition and it may often be desirable to foster the competitive spirit by separating the group into smaller groups in friendly rivalry. A ward sister once told me how she had greatly increased the morale and the work output of her ward by dividing her nurses into two groups wearing red and blue badges which she purchased in a jumble sale. She introduced a points system whereby each nurse received weekly marks on the way she had carried out her duties. The group with the higher mark at the end of each month received the ward 'cup'. Obviously the increased effort was not due to the incentive offered by the trophy but to the group spirit which was fostered by the sister's bright idea.

7. Individual Identification with the Group

Group morale will tend to be higher if each member closely identifies himself with the group. If the individual becomes absorbed in the work of the group then the group values, ideals, and principles become part of the individual's life. Anything which affects the group will equally affect the individual. Some people become so identified with a group cause that they will sacrifice a great deal, in some cases even life itself, for the group cause. There are many instances where individuals have dedicated their entire life to a group cause which has seemed to them more important and more fulfilling than personal satisfaction. Many such people, like the first Christian disciples, attain eternal fame and glory through their devotion to a cause while others, such as Adolf Hitler, achieve lasting fame of a different kind. There is, of course, a vast difference between those who put a larger cause before their personal satisfaction and those who merely use such a cause to further their own ambitions. The nursing profession certainly offers ideals and values which lead some nurses to dedicate their lives to their profession to almost the same degree as their founder, Florence Nightingale. That this is possible is salutary to professional standards and there is no doubt that the nurse who dedicates her life to nursing finds abundant compensation for her personal sacrifices. Such a nurse may also imbue her younger colleagues with some sense of the personal fulfilment to be found in nursing, particularly if she retains a wide interest in life and in people. Sometimes, however, such dedication leads to a narrowing of interest so that the individual loses touch with other aspects of life outside her work. This extreme form of identification, which replaces personality development instead of adding to it, may exert a disruptive force on the rest of the group. The dedicated nurse may lose the capacity to understand the point of view of her colleagues who have invested only part of their lives in nursing. Her colleagues in turn may be put off by the one-sidedness of her personality and fail to benefit from her experience. It is probably a mistake to narrow one's horizons too much. Nursing can be an absorbing experience but so also is living.

The nurse's identification with the group may, of course, take the less generalized form of pride in one's hospital, unit, or ward. The good ward sister will feel as involved personally in anything which happens in her ward as if it happened to her. She finds satisfaction in running an efficient and happy ward and the nurses who make up her group learn in their turn to become part of a ward team.

8. The Relationship between Group Members

Individuals are, of course, held together not only by a common identification with the group's activity but also by the personal relationships which develop between them. It is somewhat of a truism to say that morale will be higher if the group members like each other. People who get on well together work well together. Applying this principle to the hospital ward we might infer that part of the ward sister's duties, as group leader, is to minimize any personal frictions which arise between her nurses. A nurse may find it impossible to give of her best in a ward where there is a constant clash of temperament between herself and a colleague. If the underlying cause of such friction cannot be disclosed and the situation remedied it may be better for all concerned if the individuals are posted to other wards where the same conditions will not operate.

9. The Role of the Group Leader

In the previous points raised we have continually referred to the function of the group leader and there is no doubt that the state of morale of any group is intimately related to the leader's activity. With the presence of a leader, each member of the group will work not only for the group but for the approval and goodwill of the leader. Many people who have studied group behaviour believe that this is the most important feature in the stability of any group. In other words, a group may stand or fall according to the abilities and the personality of the leader. One may, again, refer to Britain in time of war for an example here when the personality and leadership qualities of Winston Churchill did more than anything to unite Britain into a stable group. In the ward group the ward sister is the natural leader and the whole atmosphere of the ward will depend in a large measure upon her personality. Nurses attain promotion according to such factors as general technical efficiency, seniority, and ability to take responsibility. These qualities are, of course, highly relevant but perhaps too little attention is sometimes paid to the nurse's capacity to guide, lead, and organize others. The question of good leadership is relevant not only to the role of the sister and other senior nurses but also to the most junior nurse who will be regarded as a figure of authority by the patients. In mental nursing, leadership is particularly important for, as we have already mentioned, the modern approach to mental illness places the nurse as the nominal leader of the patient group. Our discussion on group morale thus leads us on naturally to the related question of the factors involved in leadership.

Leadership

'He is a born leader!' This is the sort of statement one hears people make when assessing an individual's leadership qualities, the inference being that these qualities are inherent features of personality rather than acquired skills. During war-time the army authorities worked on the principle that certain people had 'the stuff of leadership' in them and it was this capacity for leadership which the officer selection boards tried to assess. It was assumed that, given the right 'officer material,' the training course would develop this raw material into the finished product of a man who could inspire confidence in others. Most of us would agree that there are some individuals who would never make good leaders while there are others who do seem to fit in with the conception of a person born to lead others. Many people who do not fit into either extreme are, however, called upon to act in the capacity of a leader and it is therefore imperative that we know something of the general functions and personal qualities involved in leadership. It is, of course, slightly artificial to speak of 'leadership' in general for the function of the leader may vary widely from one group to another. The efficient officer may later show himself unable to cope with a position of authority in his civilian work. Another person may be unsuited for the responsibility of leadership at work but make an excellent leader of a social organization. By and large, however, most forms of leadership demand certain common qualities which we will now consider. As the most obvious leader in the ward setting is the ward sister we will relate such qualities as far as possible to the sister's role.

The Qualities of Leadership

1. A Belief in the Group's Aims

As the primary role of the leader is co-ordinator of the group's activities, the leader must naturally have strong convictions regarding the aims of the group. If the group leader does not completely believe in what the group is trying to do it is unlikely that the group members will be enthusiastic about their tasks. The ward sister must have implicit faith in the work of the ward so that the nurses under her will be imbued by the same spirit of doing a worth while job. Nothing is more calculated to demoralize a ward than a sister who is half-hearted about her work.

2. Delegation of Responsibility

Co-ordination depends on an adequate system of delegation so the leader must possess the ability to delegate responsibility to others. Many people are extremely efficient at coping with work themselves but lack the ability to act in an executive role. The sister may have full control over everything going on in the ward but retain full responsibility for all decisions. If the nurses under her are merely carrying out her orders in a passive way they have no opportunity of learning to make their own decisions. The correct form of leadership should involve the training of others to act as deputy leaders who will eventually be able to take command in their own right. The sister who denies the nurses this training may still run an efficient enough ward on the surface, but she is not fulfilling her true teaching role. Lack of adequate delegation also results in the efficiency of the group falling off drastically in any situation where the group leader is absent. Nothing is more calculated to annoy the visiting doctor than a group of nurses who answer his every question with 'You will have to ask Sister about that'. Delegation, of course, demands the ability to assess which members of the group have the necessary qualities to accept responsibility, so the ward sister must be able to judge correctly the abilities of her nurses.

3. Communication

As the leader functions as the group's representative in the group's communications with others, the leader must be able to relay such communications to the group. The ward sister may forget that her nurses cannot read her mind and fail to keep the group as well informed as she is herself. She must also ensure that the information she does pass on is relayed in an undistorted way to each nurse in her ward, leaving no room for misunderstandings.

4. Specific Abilities

The good group leader usually possesses certain abilities in relation to the group task which are at a higher level than the abilities of the group members. The sister, by virtue of her training and experience, has a better grasp of nursing techniques than her less experienced staff. One of the specific abilities which the leader usually has in excess of the group is intelligence. The good group leader is invariably of a higher intelligence than the average level of the group members. Although superior intelligence is an asset it is by no means the most important quality of leadership. It might indeed prove a drawback in cases where the leader's intelligence is so high relative to the group as to prevent any real communication between them.

5. Speed of Decision Making

The successful leader is able not only to make the right decisions but to make these decisions quickly. People differ in the speed by which they reach their decisions. Although the slow thinker, who considers the pros and cons of every situation fully before acting, may base his decisions on sounder reasoning his caution is not likely to inspire confidence in others. Many situations arise where the group faces an unforeseen emergency which requires prompt action. The successful leader is able to adapt his thinking to meet the new situation, quickly survey the possible ways of meeting the situation and arrive at a decisive plan of action. At times the speed of decision will be more important than whether or not the decision made was the best possible one.

6. Self-confidence

Related to the previous point is the fact that the leader must have a high degree of confidence in his own ability and be able to transmit this confidence to the group members. The ward sister is more likely to be successful if her thinking is clear cut, decisive, and backed by obvious confidence in her ability to cope with the demands of her position. The doubtful and anxious sister who is constantly unsure of the wisdom of her ideas is not likely to win the confidence and respect of the ward. This, of course, is not to say that she should be a petty dictator whose word is law. In arriving at her decisions she will take into account the views and advice of her junior colleagues and show herself flexible enough to accept any suggestions which improve on her original plan. At the same time she must show by her confident approach to any new problem that the group can turn to her in the event of any crisis.

7. Self-consistency

In our previous discussion in Chapter 3, on the adult as a nurse, we referred to the tendency of people to project or transfer their feelings aroused by past experiences with others, on to people in the present. Our reactions to others around us are coloured by our previous experiences and this is particularly true of our reactions to authority figures. Our attitude to authority is seldom completely rational for it includes the emotions aroused by past authority figures such as parents, elder siblings, teachers, and so on. The influence of these emotional factors in the way we view authority may be so strong as to lead us to try to manipulate future authority figures into acting in accordance with our expectations. The ward sister is a natural target for such transference feelings and she may find that both her nurses and her patients at times endeavour to manoeuvre her into the role which they have unconsciously cast for her. The young nurse who has, for example, been dominated by an elder sister since childhood may react in the same submissive way to the ward sister. Her behaviour may be such as to elicit the expected aggressive reactions from the sister and thus manipulate the situation to confirm her own expectations. By remaining her objective self the sister forces the nurse to give up her immature and unrealistic view of authority. The sick patient, because of his illness, may experience again the extreme feelings of rejection which he once suffered as a child in a large family. He may become over-dependent and demanding of the sister's or nurse's attention (as he once demanded the full attention of his mother) and the sister or nurse may at first attempt to comply with these excessive demands. Soon, however, the nurse is forced to decrease the attention given to the patient because of the needs of other patients. This inevitable outcome merely confirms the patient's unconscious feelings of rejection and causes a new reaction of sulky and unco-operative behaviour. The successful leader does not allow herself to fall into such traps but, by remaining constantly herself, provides a corrective experience to the people who would unconsciously manipulate her in such ways. She gives the group a sense of security and stability by being a person who is dependable and constant in her every action. Her personality remains unaltered even when her functions as leader alter so that she is the same person in her relations with her superiors as in her relations with the nurses whom she leads.

8. Sensitivity to the Needs of Others

Before one can take charge of others successfully one must be in full charge of oneself. The efficient leader then possesses above all the type of mature self-insight which we examined in detail earlier (Chapter 3). The maturely integrated person is not only in complete command of himself but is also acutely sensitive to the needs of others. This sensitivity to the feelings of other people is undoubtedly the single quality which distinctly marks the natural leader from the leader who is externally appointed. One meets individuals who always attract others around them; who will always, no matter the situation, be the one from whom others will ask for advice and guidance. Sometimes they are not officially recognized as figures of authority and leadership but in times of crisis it is such people who become the focus of the group's faith. One of the best descriptions of this type of person is provided by Moreno in his sociometric analysis of group relations: 'They are the members (of any group) who are the most wanted participants and who have earned their choice status because they act on behalf of others with a sensitivity of response which does not characterize the average individual. They . . . see beyond the narrow circumference of their personal needs into the wide range of needs of their fellows. They are the individuals who go furthest in relating themselves to others and in translating the needs of others into effective outlets' (Moreno, 1934).

9. An Acceptance of the Responsibilities of Leadership

An individual may possess all the qualities of leadership yet have no desire to lead. A final prerequisite of the leader is then that he is willing to face the responsibilities of leadership. Unfortunately, this often means that people are appointed as leaders by virtue of their personal need to dominate others. The forceful drive of such a person may overshadow the less obvious but possibly more admirable qualities of others who are less inclined to seek positions of power. Certainly the leader must accept the power which goes with his position but, if his need to dominate others is over-pronounced, he may misuse his position merely to further his own ambitions. A need for prestige and power is often a sign of inner insecurity in that the individual is unable to relate himself to others in equal terms. There is little doubt that some neurotic and unstable people succeed to power mainly because of the very need to manipulate others which renders them most unsuited for the position of leadership. The stable leader represents the group's ends and leads by guidance, while the unstable leader represents his own ends and leads by manipulation.

We have listed here some of the personal qualities which

endow an individual with attributes of leadership. There are, of course, many other characteristics which play a part in effective leadership. The person's appearance may be highly important for others are impressed by 'strong' features, good physical stature, an attractive and forceful manner of speech, and other stereotyped characteristics which elicit confidence.

Types of Leadership

From what we have been saying of the qualities of leadership it will perhaps already be evident that there are two main forms which leadership can take. The dominating autocratic person who extracts the maximum amount of power out of his position is quite a different type of leader from the person who depends less on authority and more on his capacity to inspire others to follow him. These two main types of leadership have been termed *authoritarian* and *democratic* leadership. The authoritarian leader plans all the group activities and decides the work done by each member without consulting the group in the process. His word is law and there is no room for argument or discussion once an order has been given. He delegates only the minimum responsibility to others and actively discourages any show of initiative or independent thinking by the group members. The group is simply there to carry out the leader's orders. In contrast to this the democratic leader encourages the maximum involvement of the group in planning group activities. He delegates as much responsibility to the members as possible and acts as a co-ordinator rather than a dictator. The reasons for any decisions made by the democratic leader are explained fully to all members who are encouraged to voice their views. Most nurses will probably have experienced both authoritarian and democratic leadership and will have formed their own opinions as to their relative effectiveness. Obviously some situations will call for a more authoritarian group structure while others will be conducive to democratic leadership. Several experimental studies have, however, been carried out to examine the effects of these two types of leadership on groups working towards specific objectives.

One of the most famous of these comparative studies is that carried out by Lewin, Lippitt, and White (1939). This investigation consisted of detailed observation of a number of children's activity groups each led by an adult leader who adopted in some cases an authoritarian role and in others a democratic role. The observations showed clear differences between the two types of groups as regards their internal behaviour. The authoritarian group tended often to be more aggressive than the democratic group, the aggression being directed not towards the leader but displaced towards other members, usually those who occupied a scapegoat role in the group. Other authoritarian groups were non-aggressive but markedly apathetic. However, in the absence of the leader the apathy was replaced by internal hostility and aggression. The approaches to the leader varied between the two types of groups, that of the authoritarian group members being more submissive and often apparently merely with the object of obtaining the leader's attention rather than being positively orientated towards the group. Group unity and feelings of 'belonging' were much more evident in the democratic relative to the authoritarian group. The absence of the leader resulted in a falling off of work output in the authoritarian group while the democratic group continued with little change. When outside pressure and frustrating situations were brought to bear on the authoritarian group the result was internal hostility often leading to disintegration of the group structure. The same conditions tended to have the opposite result in the case of the democratic group, the members being more firmly united against the obstacle. Thus, in general, the democratically led type of group appears to be more cohesive and shows a higher morale than the authoritatively led group. However, the experimenters reported numerous exceptions to the general rule in that some children appeared to welcome and work best under an authoritarian leader. There was some evidence that such children came from homes showing a distinctly authoritarian structure and it would seem likely that the more insecure and unstable individual finds an authoritarian leader comforting and less anxiety provoking. I have heard the same type of comment from young nurses, some of whom become very anxious when working in a ward run on democratic lines. They prefer to be given direct orders by an authoritarian sister rather than be faced with the responsibility and insecurity of having to make their own decisions occasionally. 'Sister X may be a tartar but you know where you are with her.' A rigid régime may make fewer demands on our initiative but we are unlikely to become an efficient and self-confident person without actively participating in the group's activities. The completely authoritarian and completely democratic forms of leadership are, of course, artificial extremes. The effective leader will use her direct authority when the occasion demands it but the respect which she wins from her democratic approach to the group will ensure that such occasions seldom arise.

Assessing Leadership

In a society which depends on adequate leadership in so many fields it becomes a matter of importance to select potential leaders in the most efficient way possible. Many large industrial concerns now employ psychologists and other staff to assess candidates according to their capacity to organize others in a productive way. The methods used in such selection procedures include individual interviews, group interviews, direct observation of group behaviour, and often a battery of psychological tests designed to measure the personal abilities associated with leadership. These procedures yield most interesting and valuable information which cuts down the wastage involved in training a person to assume a position for which he is really unsuited. Qualities such as intelligence, anticipation, speed in making decisions, self-confidence, etc., can be measured fairly successfully by modern psychological testing. Other qualities, such as a sensitivity to the needs of others, are less tangible and less easily assessed. Unfortunately it is usually the qualities which prove to be most important in successful leadership which are most resistive to psychological measurement. Sometimes these qualities emerge if we compare our impression of the person in individual interview to that given by observing his behaviour as one of a group. If a number of people sit round a table to have a discussion, or join together in some form of activity, the interpersonal role of each individual may become more apparent. The able but excessively dominating person may overshadow the proceedings but only at the obvious cost of arousing the antagonism of the rest of the group. Some people will be seen to fall in habitually with the suggestions of others whom they seem over-willing to follow. An individual may, however, emerge as the natural group leader by his obvious capacity to influence the thinking and actions of the others who are willing to be guided by his views.

It is sometimes suggested that a more efficient procedure could be devised to select from nurses in training those most likely to be good candidates for later supervisory positions. There seems little doubt that the present approach to this important problem might benefit from an injection of modern selection methods. If, however, we survey the results of psychological selection in other fields we must honestly admit their limitations as well as their usefulness. At the present moment it is unlikely that traditional methods of nursing selection could be successfully supplanted by psychological assessments although some aspects of such methods of assessment would probably add to the effectiveness of current procedures.

A view one often hears expressed by nurses in relation to promotion is that 'the good nurse is seldom the successful nurses'. This view is founded on the principle that the nurse who enjoys nursing is less inclined to promotion which will involve her in supervisory duties at the expense of a great deal of direct nursing. It is true that each rung of the promotion ladder takes the nurse a little farther away from direct nursing contact with the patient. The work of the supervisory nurse is, however, no less based on nursing for she soon learns that her co-ordination and planning have a very direct effect upon the patients' welfare. In a sense she can achieve her purpose of doing more for the patient by supervizing and organizing the facilities offered by the hospital than by a close but more limited face to face relationship with her patients. It is, of course, completely understandable that some nurses find more satisfaction and reward in the direct and more intimate nurse-patient relationship which arises in general nursing duties.

Concluding Remarks

We might end this chapter by concluding that good morale and leadership are founded upon the interpersonal processes which evolve in any group. A group is not merely a number of people united by a common activity but a dynamic structure which takes its form from the relationships which exist between the group members. Each of us depends on our group relations to develop our own personality and find expression for our need to be part of something larger than ourselves. The effectiveness of any group will depend upon the degree to which it offers its members an opportunity to express themselves in working harmoniously with others. The group will fail in its function if any of its members is denied the right to participate actively in the group activities and fails to obtain the satisfaction which comes from the knowledge that one is contributing to the joint activity of living.

QUESTIONS

1. Describe some of the factors which tend to affect nursing morale. What suggestions would you make in order to maintain the ward morale at its highest level?

2. Describe the qualities which combine to make the good leader. Which of these qualities are the most important with regard to the supervisory nurse?

3. Compare the relative merits and demerits of democratic and authoritarian types of leadership. To what extent can democratic leadership operate in the setting of the hospital nursing group?

14. Group Pressure

Studies of Conformity

A middle-aged lady enters a television repair shop, carrying her portable TV. The unsmiling counter assistant explains to her that recent research has disclosed that viewing difficulties often represent a breakdown in the relationship between the viewer and the television receiver. Indeed, he continues, it has often been found to be more effective and less expensive to adjust the viewer rather than the set. If the customer will step into the rear room the mechanic will make a few minor adjustments to her which will ensure perfect viewing. The lady looks somewhat perplexed but finally asks how long it will take and if it will be painful. Reassured on both counts she agrees to the suggested procedure. The watching audience laugh at another 'Candid Camera' episode.

A psychologist stops passers-by in a busy shopping thoroughfare and asks each person if he would kindly stand on his head. The general response is to greet the request with a curious stare and walk on. A little later on the psychologist repeats his routine, but now he prefaces his strange request with a few introductory words: 'Excuse me, I am a psychologist doing research. Would you mind standing on your head?' This time about one in three of the passers-by approached agree to co-operate.

Imagine you are one of a group of adults who have been invited to take part in a three day study of the personal characteristics of people who are functioning well in their occupation. You are possibly flattered to be included in this group of bright able people who share qualities of leadership. On the last day of the study you find yourself as one of a group of five in an investigation of the accuracy of your judgements. You and your four colleagues are shown, on a series of slides, a number of problems requiring you to make simple perceptual judgements (*e.g.* which of 5 lines are equivalent in size to a standard line). The task is relatively easy and you are not at all surprised to find that your group of five are always in complete accord in their individual responses. The order of responding in the group is continually changed and eventually you find that you are the last of the five to give your response. You glance at the next slide, quickly note the correct answer and sit back confidently awaiting the response from the other four subjects before giving your own. To your amazement the first subject gives a response which is obviously incorrect. Your surprise changes to discomfort as each subject in turn indicates his agreement with the first subject. Do you stick to your guns and state your own, now deviant opinion, or go along with the group? Let's say you do back the confidence of your own judgement, only to find that this experience of being the odd man out is repeated over and over again as succeeding problems are presented. By now the other four subjects are looking at you oddly and even laughing at your responses. Your self-confidence is rapidly fading and gradually you begin to feel that the responses of your colleagues make more sense than appeared at first and that you are in agreement with them. Once this decision is made you feel much more at ease. You are again one of the group and no longer the odd outsider. Of course, you have no way of knowing that you are unwitting victim in a contrived study of conforming behaviour and that your four 'colleagues' are acting in conjunction with the experimenter.

These varied examples all provide illustrations of the degree to which people may be manipulated to behave in ways contrary to their normal individual standards. As we commented in the preceding chapter the influence of group pressures on our behaviour is normally a great deal more subtle and insidious than those evident in these illustrations. From childhood onwards we are consistently subjected to a complex set of pressures to think and behave like other members of the groups to which we belong. Such conforming behaviour ensures our acceptance within the group and the security of belongingness. Rejection of group norms and persistently individualized behaviour brings a sense of isolation and the uneasy experience of being different. Such pressures continue and perhaps intensify in adult life as we are required to 'fit-in' with the demands of various occupational, social, and recreational groups.

Another parallel problem is provided by the increasingly

complex nature of modern society, containing rapidly changing events that we often can only vaguely understand. More and more we find ourselves dependent upon the 'experts,' those individuals who are qualified to be knowledgeable about various aspects of our environment and ourselves. The physician, the scientist, the economist, the politician, the sociologist, and psychologist, and many other latter-day authorities dispense advice and wisdom on topics which seem beyond our understanding. Often there seems little choice but to hopefully accept that their pronouncements are based upon a good level of knowledge properly applied. Most of us can only hope to find a reasonable compromise between the extremes of complete rejection and uncritical acceptance of the wisdom of expert authority.

However, both everyday experience and research suggests that people vary greatly in the success with which they achieve this compromise. Some people appear to be more suggestible and more easily manipulated than others, while others are unusually resistant to such pressures. If this is so, is it simply that the more compliant are less well informed? Or, alternatively, are some people by virtue of their personality make-up more easily swayed by the crowd or by the power of authority? To attempt to answer this question we now turn to some of research studies aimed at delineating the characteristics of conforming and non-conforming persons.

Characteristics of Conformers

The first attempts to measure conforming behaviour systematically were made by psychologists such as Asch (1956) and Crutchfield (1955) using techniques similar to that described in the five man group type of experiment described in our opening examples. As might be expected, it was found that individual subjects varied greatly in terms of their conformity scores. The investigators were particularly interested in the extreme scorers, those who showed a ready tendency to be swayed by group pressure and those who consistently resisted such pressure. Further studies were carried out to examine any differences in the personality make-up of people falling into these two contrasting groups.

Such assessments did demonstrate certain fairly well defined patterns differentiating the two groups. Those subjects who returned high scores on the group tests (over-conformers) tended to be overly-accepting, submissive people in their everyday behaviour. They displayed a rather narrow range of interests, tended to be inhibited and rigid, slow and vacillating in decision making, confused and disorganized under stress, over anxious and over reponsive to the evaluations of others. In vivid contrast to this profile, the low scorers on the group tests (non-conformers) were more likely to be described as efficient, capable, self-reliant and persuasive. They were seen as good leaders and as the sort of person others would turn to for advice. Although active and vigorous in their work and hobbies, they were also regarded as natural, unaffected and relaxed. Where the subjects were themselves parents, the conformers tended to be rather restrictive with their children, while the non-conformers were more permissive.

It would thus appear that certain types of personality are more easily manipulated by group pressures than others. However, the position is probably a great deal more complicated than this analysis suggests. Other studies of suggestibility demonstrate that normally non-suggestible individuals may conform to a surprising degree in specific social situations which cause them to be more vulnerable.

Conformity to Authority

The first two illustrations of conformity with which we opened this chapter contained an element additional to the impact of group pressure upon the individual. The lady in the television repair shop unquestionably accepted the authority and expertise of the mechanic, while the strange request made of the passers-by in the second illustration gained substance by being made by a 'research psychologist'.

It might be anticipated that the probability of conformity to suggestion would be greater if the suggestion is made by someone who is regarded as a responsible authority figure.

We have already commented upon the dangers of a too-ready willingness to shelve our individual responsibility for our actions by blindly obeying others. How far will people go in acceding to the dictates of authority, particularly when they are being urged to act in ways contrary to their own moral standards? This becomes an acute question in times of war when the conflict between obeying the orders of superiors and following the dictates of one's own conscience may be repeatedly evident. For example, to what extent can the guards at Auschwitz, the rank and file soldier in Vietnam, or the airman who releases the bomb which will kill and maim, be held responsible for the misery resulting from their allegiance to orders from above?

It was precisely with these questions in mind that a psychologist called Stanley Milgram (1963) conducted an unusual and rather frightening series of experiments in the 1960's. Milgram advertised for a number of male adults to take part as paid subjects in an experiment on the effect of punishment on memory. Subjects were instructed that they would work in pairs, one as 'teacher' and one as 'pupil'. The pupil would be strapped in an 'electric chair' apparatus in a small booth and be required to answer questions on a learning test put to him by the subject acting as the teacher. Each time the pupil gave an incorrect response or did not respond to a test question, the teacher was asked to press a button giving the pupil an electric shock. The teachers were told by Milgram that the punishment must be progressively increased by the teacher raising the voltage given for each successive error by manipulating a lever in front of him. The lever could be moved among 30 positions each clearly marked with the appropriate voltage (from 15 to 450 volts) clearly designated as 'Slight Shock,' 'Danger Severe Shock,' etc. As the experiment went on the victims' protests and screams were clearly audible. Some victims referred to their having a heart condition while being strapped into the apparatus. After reaching the 300 volt level there was an ominous silence from the victim who had been banging on the booth and protesting about the pain a few minutes before. When this happened, the teacher was told by Milgram to continue with the assigned items, increasing shock intensity each time there was no response from the victims.

Before conducting the experiment, Milgram presented his plan to a large group of psychology students and asked them to estimate what proportion of 100 adults would be likely to obey all instructions and continue to the end of the experiment, thereby giving a dangerous 450 volt shock to their victim. The class estimates varied between 0 and 3 per cent with the average guess predicting that only about 1 in 100 subjects would conform to all instructions. Milgram then proceeded with his experiment and found that 65 per cent of his subjects complied with all instructions. Before the reader concludes that this experiment illustrates the sadistic tendencies of research psychologists, let me hasten to explain that the situation was completely contrived. The pupil in each case was really a confederate of Milgram's posing as a subject and of course, he was not receiving actual shocks. However, the true subjects who acted as teachers did not know this.

How does one interpret these findings? Can we preserve our faith in human nature by assuming that, for some reason, Milgram had been unfortunate enough to have unwittingly recruited a goodly number of cold-blooded psychopaths in his group of subjects? This explanation seems unlikely in that these subjects who did continue to administer severe punishment according to instructions were obviously extremely upset by the experiment which they found traumatic and about as harrowing as their imagined victim. Describing the reactions of one of his teacher subjects Milgram declares:

'I observed a mature and initially poised businessman enter the laboratory smiling and confident. Within 20 minutes he was reduced to a twitching, stuttering wreck, who was rapidly approaching a point of nervous collapse. He constantly pulled on his earlobe, and twisted his hands. At one point he pushed his fist in his forehead and muttered "Oh, God, let's stop it," and yet he continued to respond to every word of the experimenter and obeyed to the end.'

Obviously most of the teacher subjects felt compelled to act in a manner contrary, not only to the interests of their pupil, but also to their own personal dictates. Why then did they continue to obey the instructions? Milgram deduced that a prime factor in this situation was the authority engendered by the fact that the experimenter was a professor of psychology at a respectable university (Yale). There seems little doubt that the unquestioning acceptance of the suggestions of an apparently reliable authority figure is a powerful force in the readiness with which people will perform actions normally regarded as anti-social. In his study of the efficacy of hypnosis in evoking anti-social behaviour, Barber (1969) instructed non-hypnotized subjects to throw a liquid, described as highly corrosive acid (but actually a harmless fluid) over a fellow subject. The substantial proportion who obeyed the instructions later justified their ostensibly anti-social behaviour on the grounds that the status of the experimenter made it unlikely that he would risk any severe bodily harm to his subjects. It should, however, be made plain that Milgram's subjects were fully convinced, at the time of the experiment, that the shocks they administered to their victims were genuine.

In a later study Milgram (1964) examined the outcome in a similar situation where the effect of obedience to an authority figure was replaced by that of peer group pressure. Here the true subject found himself to be one of a group of three 'teachers,' the other two of whom were again confederates of Milgram. Each group of three were told that each member would vote in turn on the level of shock to be administered to the pupil each time he made an error in the learning test. However, the actual shock value to be given would be that corresponding to the lowest intensity suggested by any member of the three man group. The procedure was manipulated so that the true subject always voted last, after the two confederates each in turn suggested an increase in shock value for each trial. The true subject then had in effect the casting vote, in that the instructions allowed him to overrule the two preceding votes and maintain the shocks at a low level. Milgram also ran a parallel control situation in which the true subject was the sole arbitrator in deciding the intensity of shock to be given after each error.

The tendency was for the subject to reach a compromise reaction to group pressure by opting for shock values roughly half-way between the high intensities suggested by his peer group and those he would advocate himself in the absence of peer group pressure. In other words, the effect of peer group pressure in inducing this form of anti-social behaviour was somewhat less than that induced by the authority effect, but still nevertheless clearly evident.

I have described Milgram's work in some detail because it provides a very vivid illustration of the degree to which many people are prepared to accept the dictates of authoritarian or group pressure. Milgram saw his study as a miniscule demonstration of the denial of self responsibility which can occur in a much more dramatic fashion in times of war and social unrest. People of any nation, at any time, he argues, may be fairly easily manipulated by the pressure of society to behave in a manner alien to their individual moral code. Comparatively recent world events have made Milgram's suggestion of even grimmer import.

At this point the reader may well wonder to what extent such conforming anti-social behaviour might be modified by the fellow-feeling induced by some form of kinship between the victim and his persecutor. Milgram's subjects were unknown to each other. Might they be less likely to obey instructions which would imperil someone who was less anonymous and known to them?

The likelihood of this suggestion is heightened by another study (Zimbardo, 1969). Here student volunteers were assigned to four person groups. In one type of group the subjects were rendered as anonymous as possible by being shrouded in bulky coats and hoods. Subjects in the other groups were clearly visible, wore name tags and were frequently referred to by name by the experimenter. Both groups were placed in an experimental condition which ostensibly involved their giving painful electric shocks to two girls who were confederates of the experimenter. It was found that the subjects in the anonymous condition were much more aggressive, giving stronger shocks, than the subjects in the individualized groups. This study demonstrates that anonymity has a heightening effect in the perpetration of aggressive acts upon others, whereas an underlining of personal identity and individuation lowers the likelihood of such behaviour. Milgram (1965) found a similar effect in another study in which he systematically varied the closeness of the relationship between the teacher subjects and their victims. His findings clearly demonstrated a lessening of obedience to instructions as the proximity of aggressor and victim increased. It is somewhat alarming to note that even in the condition of closest proximity, in which the subject was required to hold his protesting victim's arm down on the shock pad while administering the shocks, approximately one in every three subjects still obeyed all instructions.

One effective method of increasing the anonymity of the victim, (and thus increasing the likelihood of people conforming to aggressive instructions), is to have the victim appear as alien, sub-human, and in different ways less deserving of humane behaviour. This, of course, is exactly what the propaganda machines of wartime seek to do to our perception of the enemy we must learn to kill without guilt or compunction. However, the strategies used to evoke such conforming behaviour are by no means limited to international conflict.

Most civilized people reacted with abhorrence to Hitler's so-called Final Solution to the 'Jewish problem' in Nazi Germany. In 1969 a social scientist at the University of Hawaii (Mansson, 1969) assembled over 500 students to seek their co-operation in a scientific project to solve 'the problem of the mentally ill and emotionally unfit'. The students were given a long authoritative discourse upon the increasingly higher rate of breeding in the mentally and emotionally unfit members of the population, who might eventually endanger the fit segment of society. It was suggested that the only feasible solution was a legalized and widespread programme of euthanasia or mercy killing. It was emphasized that this extermination of the unfit would be both a boon to healthy mankind and a kindness to the (sub-human) mentally unfit. Presented with this parallel solution to Hitler's programme, (but couched as a respectable scientific programme) just over two thirds of the 500 students indicated their approval of this programme of 'systematic killing'. Another thought-provoking illustration of the effects of relatively unsubtle pressures upon individual standards of conduct.

Concluding Remarks

Almost from the moment of birth, each of us is subjected to a variety of pressures, some direct, others more subtle, from the society of which we are a part. In this chapter we have seen how some of these group pressures may influence our individual behaviour, without us necessarily being aware of their effect upon us. Some people would appear to be particularly susceptible to such group pressures by virtue of their over-conforming personality make-up. The tendency to be swayed by our adherence to the views of authority figures heightens the likelihood of conforming behaviour and we have considered some of the unfortunate results which may emerge from us resigning our individual sense of responsibility in favour of authority.

It may be worth adding here that, although we have dwelt primarily upon somewhat negative and anti-social results of group pressures, there is no reason why such pressures should not be as efficiently utilized towards positive and socialized behaviours.

QUESTIONS

1. Describe techniques used to measure individual differences in conformity.

2. Comment upon some of the factors which effect individual response to obeying authority.

Summary and Conclusion

In the preceding chapters an attempt has been made to acquaint the nurse with some aspects of human behaviour seen from a psychological viewpoint. We have examined first some of the many factors which influence our development from infancy to old age and help to shape our personality. In the second part of the book we have dealt briefly with some of the forces which motivate us in our individual behaviour and we have discussed in broad outline the relative contributions of heredity and environment in making us what we are. The third part of our discussion led us to a brief description of the different processes by which we react to our environment and accumulate the knowledge arising from our experiences. Finally we have reminded ourselves that, although each of us is a separate individual, we develop our personality and attain personal fulfilment only in our capacity to relate ourselves to others. We are essentially social beings whose happiness is dependent upon establishing harmonious relations with others in the groups of which we are a part.

I have tried to demonstrate some of the findings of psychological investigations of human behaviour and to evaluate these facts as fairly as possible. Every book is, however, limited by the personal convictions of its author and the psychologist is certainly not immune from the tendency to select the material which suits his own orientation and general outlook. Throughout the preceding chapters there are at least two broad themes which betray the convictions of the present author and it is these general principles I would like to leave in the reader's mind. I have repeatedly stressed the view that each individual owes it to himself to become what is in him to become. We are each of us born as individuals with inherent possibilities which often remain undeveloped due to the self-limiting restrictions we place upon ourselves. Certain limitations are imposed on us by inheritance and unavoidable circumstances but the wide scope left for development is seldom explored due to lack of confidence, over-dependence on the opinion of others, sheer apathy and other inner restrictions which prevent us expressing ourselves fully. The more insight we develop into the nature of our limitations and potentialities the more free we become to expand our sphere of living beyond the artificial boundaries set by immaturity, ignorance, and fear. An appreciation of some of the processes controlling human behaviour can aid us in accepting ourselves as independent individuals and also teach us to understand and accept the integrity of others. It is sometimes said that we have a moral duty to help others. In actual fact, it is only through our love and acceptance of others that we come to know more of our own self and find a mature satisfaction in living. This is true whether we are referring to friendship, marriage, every-day social interaction, or work. Each of these experiences will be richer if we learn to dispense with the need for self-deception and the tendency to manipulate others to suit our own purposes.

The other general theme which has been constantly emphasized is that we tend to exaggerate the rational nature of human behaviour. If our conduct were always guided by reason life would be much less complicated (although perhaps less exciting) and human behaviour much more predictable. As it is, our behaviour is influenced by a variety of forces, many of which lie outside our immediate awareness. We have seen that the irrational thinking of the emotionally disturbed or mentally ill patient provides only an exaggerated picture of the illogical nature of much normal adult thinking. An appreciation of this aspect of our thinking allows us to guard against some of the subjective bias which may colour our thinking and prevent us dealing with our environment in an objective and reasonable manner.

Finally, let us try to justify the title of this book by questioning its relevance to nursing. Any addition to an already overloaded training curriculum is liable to be greeted with distaste by the student nurse who must feel that she will be a walking encyclopedia by the time she qualifies. Unfortunately her patients will bring with them into hospital not only their illness but their whole personality. The way the patients think and feel about their present situation, their past experiences, and their view of the future, will all combine to influence their behaviour in hospital and the way they will react to their illness. The nurse who has some appreciation of the factors involved will be better equipped to aid the patient as effectively as possible. The nurse is also a representative of a profession to which the public turn for guidance and information. In this capacity as an authoritative expert on human health it would seem essential that the nurse have some idea of the psychological side of development. A third justification for the time and energy demanded by learning something of psychology is the optimistic assumption that the reader may find something in these pages which interests her as a person and opens her mind to new possibilities.

In our introduction we differentiated psychological study from the 'commonsense' observation of human behaviour by saying that the former tried to arrive at its conclusions in as objective and scientific a manner as possible. However, no one can ever call themselves an expert in the study of human behaviour. Each of you, by virtue of your working role as a nurse, studies human behaviour every minute of the day. Some of the ideas expressed here may aid you in becoming a better observer of others and may also help in the first job of understanding yourself to a better degree. However, in the field of human behaviour there is no clear right and wrong such as, for example, in the field of mathematics. If this book only has the result of making you think a little critically about the ideas expressed, even if you arrive at independent and contrary conclusions, then it will have had some point. Psychology is a young science. It has much to learn and often those who write about it are people who could well do with spending less time writing and more time mixing with people and endeavouring to understand their problems. In summary, then, it is hoped that you will have understood and, in some ways, appreciated what you have read, but it is also hoped that you will not passively accept every statement without further thought. I trust instead that what has been said will stimulate you to question the basis of your own experience and arrive at the independent and personal judgment which you have every right to make and for which your job as a nurse aptly qualifies you.

Successful teaching becomes successful only at the point where the student begins to question the ideas and conclusions of his teacher.

Glossary

A short explanation is given below of a few of the terms used in the text which may be unfamiliar to the reader. This glossary is confined to terms which have not already been defined and explained in the text of the book itself. It has been compiled with the aid of Warren's *Dictionary of Psychology*, the dictionary definition being quoted in cases where the meaning of the term is at all ambiguous.

1. **Adaptability.** The ability of an individual to make successful adjustments to changes in his general environment.
2. **Adualism.** The term used by genetic psychologists such as Piaget to describe the stage of infantile development during the first seven or eight months of life. The main characteristic of this stage is a lack of differentiation between internal mentality and external reality. There is thus, during this phase of development, no differentiation between the self and the outside world, no awareness, and no capacity to form a relationship with external objects or people.
3. **Affect.** An inclusive term used to denote any variety of emotional experiences or moods.
4. **Ambivalence.** The holding of contradictory or opposite feelings (usually feelings of love and hate) towards the same person.
5. **Anthropology.** Anthropology as a whole includes all the sciences which investigate the human species. The more specific branch of anthropology to which we have referred in the text is social anthropology, which studies the similarities and differences between societies and the types of social relationships which are formed in different societies.
6. **Constitution.** This term is used to indicate that part of the individual's personality which is basically inborn, inherited, and present, although sometimes in a latent form from birth. This is in marked distinction to the psychogenic or environmental attributes of personality which are developed as a result of the impact and experience and learning on the individual. The distinction between these two terms is somewhat false in that all

constitutional factors are acted upon and their development influenced by the environment.

7. **Depersonalization.** Describes the sensation of unreality, where one's self or one's own body is experienced as being strange or unfamiliar. An allied term *derealization* describes a similar experience where objects and events in the outside world are perceived as being strange, unreal, and unfamiliar. These allied experiences are a common feature of any mental disorder in which acute anxiety is present, but they are also experienced as a transitory phenomenon in normal subjects in times of stress.
8. **Deterioration.** An impairment of mental function or of personality. Intellectual deterioration is a term usually used to describe an abnormal degree of deterioration in an individual's intellectual capacity outwith that which one would expect through the normal process of ageing.
9. **Electro-encephalogram** (EEG). The apparatus which is used to obtain amplified readings of the electro-chemical discharges of the brain. These discharges are translated by the apparatus into a pen recorded trace which represents certain characteristics of the electrical activity in different regions of the brain. The EEG is principally used as a means of diagnosing disorders of the brain and nervous system, such as epilepsy.
10. **Endogenous.** This term is used to describe mental symptoms which arise from internal (e.g., biochemical) changes in the body, as opposed to symptoms which arise through the individual's reactions to environmental events, these latter symptoms being referred to as exogenous or psychogenically determined.
11. **Egocentric.** A person is described as egocentric when he responds to all situations from a personal viewpoint. The term means literally 'selfcentred'. It is used by genetic psychologists, such as Piaget, to describe the nature of the child's thinking and to differentiate it from adult thinking which is more objective and orientated towards the outside world.
12. **Environment.** This is a general term embracing all stimuli which, although external to the individual, affect his behaviour. It usually refers particularly to all objects and persons with whom the individual comes into some form of social contact.
13. **Ergograph.** An instrument for measuring changes in the amount of muscular contraction, usually used by experimental psychologists to measure the effects of fatigue. The usual arrangement is for the subject's hand to be strapped to a board leaving only one free finger by which the subject is asked to lift a hanging weight repeatedly. A record of the subject's performance is made on a graph which illustrates his working capacity over a period of time.
14. **Extraversion.** The type of personality in which the individual's interests are directed mainly towards the external environment and other people, rather than towards the individual's inner experiences.

15. **Factor Analysis.** A statistical technique which attempts to extract from any group of measurements basic factors common to them all.
16. **Heredity.** Those basic aspects of the personality which are determined by transmission through the genes and which account for some of the resemblances of offspring to parents or their ancestors.
17. **Hypnagogic State.** The state of mind which exists immediately prior to sleep where there is a blurring of the distinction between what is imagined and what is real.
18. **Identification.** An unconscious mental process which expresses itself in the form of an emotional tie with other people in which the individual behaves as if he were the person with whom he has this tie. This is one of the basic processes in childhood learning as the child imitates and strives to be like parents and other figures in his early environment.
19. **Image.** An experience which reproduces or copies in part, and with some degree of realism, a previous perceptual experience in the absence of the original sensory stimulation. The term is usually related to memory images of past events but we may, of course, conjure up images in our mind of events or objects which we have not experienced. Images can take several forms; visual images are reproductions of visual experiences; auditory images relate to verbal experiences; gustatory images describe images of taste; olfactory images describe reproductions of smells or odours; tactile images relate to reproductions of sensations of touch; and kinaesthetic images describe images of bodily movement.
20. **Innate.** This adjective describes any capacity or ability which is present in the individual at birth. Although inherited and present at birth, an innately determined response may not show itself in behaviour until later in childhood. When this is the case it is said that maturation has occurred in that the response could not operate until the neural pathways in the brain had developed during the post-natal life.
21. **Intellectual Capacity.** This term describes the abilities which we are capable of developing and is contrasted with *mental ability* which refers to the abilities which have been developed. Thus a person may have a high intellectual capacity but because of circumstances this capacity may remain undeveloped so that he has a poor intellectual ability.
22. **Introversion.** The type of personality in which the individual's interests are turned inward towards himself, rather than outward towards his external environment (opposite to extraversion).
23. **Neurosis.** This term usually describes mental disturbance where the individual retains contact with reality. The term is contrasted with the more serious type of mental disturbance, the

Psychoses (insanity), where the individual loses contact with reality.

24. **Objective.** Something which is localized outside the observer's body and is not dependent upon any special bias or judgment of the individual observer. This is in contrast to a subjective experience which is influenced by the individual's own internal feelings.
25. **Perception.** The process by which we become aware of objects in our environment and assign to them a meaning and significance.
26. **Phobia.** An exaggerated and pathological dread of certain specific types of stimuli or situation (e.g., *claustrophobia*—fear of being closed in).
27. **Psychotherapy.** The psychological treatment of mental disturbance where the main emphasis is on the personal relationship established between the psychotherapist and the patient. The term is used in psychiatry to contrast this form of treatment with physical methods of treatment such as electro-convulsive therapy, insulin coma therapy, etc.
28. **Reliability.** Refers in general to the dependability and accuracy of any event. This term tends to be used, however, with specific reference to psychological tests to denote the self-consistency of a test.
29. **Sensory.** Any activity which involves sensations transmitted to the brain and nervous system through separate receptors or sense organs of the body.
30. **Standardization.** The basic procedure in devising psychological tests which leads to the establishment of a fixed or standard procedure in the giving and coring of tests as well as the establishment of adequate norms.
31. **Stimulus.** Any external or internal event which alters our experience and causes us to respond in a particular way.
32. **Trauma.** An emotional shock, usually of a severe nature.
33. **Validity.** The test as to whether a psychological test is truthfully measuring that which it sets out to measure.

Bibliography

ALLPORT, G. W. (1937). *Personality*. London: Constable.

AMES, A. (1953). Reconsideration of the origin and nature of perception. In *Vision and Action*, edited by S. Ratnor. New Brunswick: Rutgers University Press.

ANTHONY, E. J. (1957). An experimental approach to psychopathology and childhood encopresis. *British Journal of Medical Psychology*, **30,** 129.

ASCH, S. E. (1956). Studies of Independence and Conformity. *A Minority of One Against a Unanimous Majority*. Psychological Monographs: General and Applied.

AYLLON, T. & MICHAEL, J. (1959). The psychiatric nurse as a behavioural engineer. *Journal of the Experimental Analysis of Behaviour*, **2,** 323.

AZRIN, N. H. & LINDSLEY, O. R. (1956). The reinforcement of cooperation between children. *Journal of Abnormal and Social Psychology*, **52,** 100.

BARBER, T. X. (1969). *Hypnosis: A Scientific Approach*. New York: Van Nostrand.

BARRON, F. (1963). *Creativity and Psychological Health*. Princeton, N.Y.: Van Nostrand.

BARRON, F. (1972). The creative personality: Akin to madness. *Psychology Today*, **6,** 2, 42.

BERGER, R. J. (1963). Dream content, experimental modification by meaningful verbal stimuli. *British Journal of Psychiatry*, **109,** 722.

BICKFORD, J. A. R. (1955). The forgotten patient. *Lancet*, **2,** 969.

BIRCH, H. G. & LEFFORD, A. (1963). Intersensory development in children. *Monographs of the Society for Research in Child Development*, **28,** 5.

BIRCH, H. G. & LEFFORD, A. (1967). Visual differentiation, intersensory integration and voluntary motor control. *Monographs of the Society for Research in Child Development*, **32,** 1.

BOWLBY, J. (1951). Maternal care and mental health. *World Health Organization Monographs*, **2.** Geneva.

BOWLBY, J., AINSWORTH, M., BOSTON, M., & ROSENBLUTH, D. (1956).

The effects of mother-child separation: a follow-up study. *British Journal of Medical Psychology*, **29**, 211.

BROADBENT, D. E. & HERON, A. (1962). Effects of a subsidiary task on performance involving immediate memory by younger and older subjects. *British Journal of Psychology*, **53**, 189.

CAMERON, J. L., LAING, R. D. & MCGHIE, A. (1955). Patient and nurse. *Lancet*, **2**, 1384.

COELHO, G. V., HAMBURG, D. A. & MURPHEY, E. B. (1963). Coping strategies in a new learning environment: A study of American College Freshmen. *Archives of General Psychiatry*, **9**, 433.

CRUTCHFIELD, R. S. (1955). Conformity and character. *American Psychologist*, **10**, 191.

DOMINIAN, J. (1968). *Marital Breakdown*. London: Penguin Books, Ltd.

DYKES, M. & MCGHIE, A. (1976). A comparative study of attentional strategies of schizophrenic and highly creative normal subjects. *British Journal of Psychiatry*, **128**, 50.

FEIFEL, H. (1959). Attitudes toward death in some normal and mentally ill populations, in *The Meaning of Death*, Ed. Feifel, H. New York, McGraw-Hill.

FLETCHER, R. (1957). *Instinct in Man*. London: Allen & Unwin.

FREUD, S. (1923). *The Ego and the Id*. London: Hogarth.

GETZELS, J. W. & JACKSON, P. W. (1962). *Creativity and Intelligence: Explorations with Gifted Students*. New York: Wiley.

GILBERTSTEN, V. A. & WANGENSTEEN, O. H. (1961). Should the doctor tell the patient that the disease is cancer? In *The Physician and the Total Care of the Cancer Patient*. New York: American Cancer Society.

GOLDMAN-EISLER, F. (1956). The determinants of the rate of speech output and their mutual relations. *Journal of Psychosomatic Research*, **1**, 137.

GOLDMAN-EISLER, F. (1958). Speech production and predictability of words in context and the length of pauses in speech. *Language and Speech*, **1**, 96.

GOLDMAN-EISLER, F. (1961). Hesitation and information in speech. In *Information Theory: Proceedings of the Fourth London Symposium on Information Theory*, p. 162. London.

GRINKER, R. R. (1962). 'Mentally Healthy young males (homoclites). *Archives of General Psychiatry*, **6**, 405.

HEBB, D. O. (1949). *Organisation of Behaviour*. London: Chapman & Hall.

HEBB, D. O. (1955). The mammal and his environment. *American Journal of Psychiatry*, **111**, 826.

HINTON, J. (1967). *Dying*. London: Penguin Books Ltd.

HYTTEN, F. E., YORSTON, J. C. & THOMSON, A. M. (1958). Difficulties associated with breast feeding: a study of 106 primiparae. *British Medical Journal*.

INGLIS, J. (1956). Immediate memory, age and brain function. In *Behaviour Aging and the Nervous System*, edited by A. T. Welford & J. E. Birren. Springfield Ill.: Thomas.

IRWIN, O. C. (1930). The amount and nature of activities of newborn infants under constant external stimulating conditions during the first ten days of life. *Genetic Psychology Monographs*, **8,** 1.

JOHNS, J. H. & QUAY, H. C. (1962). The effect of social reward on verbal conditions in psychopathic and neurotic military offenders. *Journal of Consulting Psychology*, **26,** 217.

JONES, M. C. (1924). A laboratory study of fear: The case of Peter. *Pedagogical Seminary and Journal of Genetic Psychology*, **31,** 308.

KALLMAN, F. J. (1946). The genetic theory of schizophrenia. *American Journal of Psychiatry* **13,** 309.

KAZDIN, A. E. (1975). *Behaviour Modification in Applied Settings*. London: Irwin-Dorsey.

KIMURA, D. (1960). Visual and auditory perception after temporal lobe damage. *Doctoral Thesis*, unpublished. Montreal, McGill University.

KIMURA, D. (1961). Some effects of temporal lobe damage on auditory perception. *Canadian Journal of Psychology*, **15,** 166.

KINSEY, A. C., POMEROY, W. B. & MARTIN, C. E. (1948). *Sexual Behaviour in the Human Male*. Philadelphia: Saunders.

KOHLER, I. (1961). On the development and transformation of the perceptual world. *Psychology*, **2,** 8, 193.

KOLVIN, I., OUNSTED, C., HUMPHREY, M., MCNAY, A., RICHARDSON, L., GARSIDE, R. F., KIDD, J. J. H. & ROTH, M. (1971). Studies in childhood psychoses. *British Journal of Psychiatry*, **118,** 381.

KREITMAN, N., COLLINS, J., NELSON, B. & TROOP, J. (1970). Neurosis and marital interaction: I. Personality and symptoms. *British Journal of Psychiatry*, **117,** 33.

LACEY, J. I., BATEMAN, D. E. & VAN LEHM, R. (1953). Autonomic response specificity. *Psychosomatic Medicine*, **15,** 8.

LAZARUS, R. S. (1969). *Patterns of Adjustment and Human Effectiveness*. New York: McGraw-Hill.

LEWIN, K., LIPPITT, R. & WHITE, R. K. (1939). Patterns of aggressive behaviour in experimentally created 'social climates'. *Journal of Social Psychology*, **10,** 271.

LILLY, J. C. (1956). *Psychiatric Research Report*, **1.**

LORENZ, K. (1952). *King Solomon's Ring*. London: Methuen. (Also published in Pan Books Series, 1957.)

LOWE, G. R. (1966). Response inhibition and deviant social behaviour in children. *British Journal of Psychiatry*, **112,** 925.

LURIA, A. R. (1961). *The Role of Speech in the Regulation of Normal and Abnormal Behaviour*. London: Pergamon Press.

MCDOUGALL, WM. (1933). *The Energies of Men*. New York: Scribners.

MCGHIE, A. (1957). The role of the mental nurse. *Nursing Mirror*, 17th, 24th, 31st May, and 7th June, 1957.

MCGHIE, A. (1965). Psychological studies of schizophrenia. In *Studies on Psychosis*, edited by T. Freeman, J. L. Cameron & A. McGhie. London: Tavistock Publications.

MCGHIE, A. & CHAPMAN, J. (1961). Disorders of attention and perception in early schizophrenia. *British Journal of Medical Psychology*, **34,** 103.

MCGHIE, A. & CHAPMAN, J. (1962). A comparative study of disordered attention in schizophrenia. *Journal of Mental Science*, **108**, 455, 487.

McGhie, A. & Russell, S. M. (1962). The subjective assessment of normal sleep patterns. *Journal of Mental Science*, **108**, 456.

McGhie, A., Chapman, J. & Lawson, J. S. (1965). Changes in immediate memory with age. *British Journal of Psychology*, **56**, 1, 69.

McGhie, A. & Chapman, J. (1962). A comparative study of distraction on schizophrenic performance. 1. Perception and immediate memory. *British Journal of Psychiatry*, **111**, 383.

McGhie, A., Chapman, J. & Lawson, J. S. (1965 *b*). The effect of distraction on schizophrenic performance. 2. Psychomotor ability. *British Journal of Psychiatry*, **111**, 391.

McKenzie, N. (1945). The personality of the student nurse. *In* Temperament, character, and personality. *Nursing Times*, April, May, 1945.

MacMurray, J. (1950). *Conditions of Freedom*. London: Faber.

Malmo, R. B. & Shagass, C. (1952). Studies of blood pressure in psychiatric patients under stress. *Psychosomatic Medicine*, **14**, 82.

Mandler,, A., Mandler, J. M. & Uviller, E. T. (1958). Autonomic feed back; the perception of autonomic activity. *Journal of Abnormal and Social Psychology*, **56**, 367.

Mansson, H. H. (1969). Justifying the final solution. Paper presented at the International Congress of Psychology, London. 70, 9, 416.

Masters, W. H. & Johnson, D. E. (1966). *Human Sexual Response*. London: Churchill.

Mead, Margaret (1935). *Sex and Temperament in Three Primitive Societies*. London: Routledge.

Mendelson, J. & Foley, J. (1956). *Transactions of the American Neurological Association*, **81**, 134.

Metcalfe, M. (1956). Demonstration of a psychosomatic relationship. *British Journal of Medical Psychology*, **29**, 63.

Milgram, S. (1963). Behavioural study of obedience. *Journal of Abnormal and Social Psychology*, **67**, 371.

Milgram, S. (1964). Group pressure and action against a person. *Journal of Abnormal and Social Psychology*, **69**, 137.

Milgram, S. (1965). Some conditions of obedience and disobedience to authority. *Human Relations*, **18**, 57.

Milner, B. (1958). Psychological defects produced by temporal lobe excision. *Research Publications. Association for Research in Nervous and Mental Diseases*, **36**, 244.

Milner, B. (1960). Impairment of visual recognition and recall after right temporal lobectomy in man. (Paper read at First Annual Meeting of Psychonomic Society.)

Mirsky, I. A. (1958). Physiologic, psychologic and social determinants in the aetiology of duodenal ulcers. *American Journal of Digestive Diseases*, **3**, 285.

Money, J., Hampson, J. G. & Hampson, J. L. (1957). Imprinting and the establishment of gender role. *A.M.A. Archives of Neurology and Psychiatry*, **77**, 333.

MORENO, J. L. (1934). Who shall survive? *Nervous and Mental Diseases Monograph*, **58.**

NELSON, B., COLLINS, J., KREITMAN, N. & TROOP, J. (1970). Neurosis and marital interaction. II. Time sharing and social activity. *British Journal of Psychiatry*, **117,** 47.

ODLUM, DORIS (1954). *Psychology, the Nurse and the Patient*. London: The Nursing Mirror Ltd.

ORLANSKY (1949). Infant care and personality. *Psychological Bulletin*, **46,** 1.

OSWALD, I. (1960). Falling asleep open-eyed during intense rhythmic stimulation. *British Medical Journal*, **1,** 1450.

PARKER, T. & ALLERTON, R. (1962). *The Courage of his Convictions*. London: Hutchinson.

PAYNE, R. W. & HEWLETT, J. H. G. (1960). Thought disorder in psychotic patients. In *Experiments in Personality*, ed. Eysenck, H. J. London: Routledge and Kegan Paul.

PENFIELD, W. & JASPER, H. H. (1954). *Epilepsy and the Functional Anatomy of the Human Brain*. Boston: Little, Brown & Co.

PETERSON, C. H. & SPANO, F. L. (1941). Breast feeding, maternal rejection, and child personality. *Character and Personality*, **10,** 62.

PAIGET, J. (1928). *Judgment and Reasoning in the Child*. London: Routledge and Kegan Paul.

PIAGET, J. (1932). *The Language and Thought of the Child*. London: Routledge and Kegan Paul.

PIAGET, J. (1951). *Play, Dreams, and Imitation in Childhood*. London: Heinemann.

RAVEN, J. C. (1950). A comparative assessment of personality. *British Journal of Psychology*, **40,** 115.

RAVEN, J. C. (1952). *Human Nature*. London: H. K. Lewis.

RICHMOND, J. B. & LUSTMAN, L. M. (1955). Autonomic function in the neonate: 1) Implications for psychosomatic theory. *Psychosomatic Medicine*, **17,** 269.

ROBINS, L. M. (1966). *Deviant Children Grow up*. Balitmore: Williams & Wilkins.

ROGERSON, B. C. F. & ROGERSON, C. H. (1939). Feeding in infancy and subsequent psychological difficulties. *Journal of Mental Science*, **85,** 1, 163.

ROSENHAN, D. L. (1973). On being sane in insane places. *Science*, **179,** 250.

ROSS, T. A. (1923). *The Common Neuroses*. London: Arnold & Co.

RUTTER, M. & LOCKYER, L. (1967). A five to fifteen year follow-up study of infantile psychosis. *British Journal of Psychiatry*, **113,** 1183.

SCHACHTER, S. & SINGER, J. E. (1962). Cognitive, social and physiological determinants of emotional state. *Psychological Review*, **69,** 379.

SCHAFFER, H. R. (1957). Psychological factors in the care of the child in hospital. *Nursing Mirror*, 20th, 27th Sept., 4th Oct., 1957.

SCHAFFER, H. R. (1961). Some issues for research in the study of attachment behaviour. Research report given at second Tavistock Study Group on Mother-Infant Interaction.

SCHONFIELD, M. (1968). *The Sexual Behaviour of Young People*. London: Penguin Books, Ltd.

SEARS, R. R., PINTLER, M. H. & SEARS, P. S. (1946). Effect of further separation on pre-school children's doll play aggression. *Child Development*, **17,** 219.

SEDMAN, G. (1966). A comparative study of pseudohallucinations, imagery and true hallucinations. *British Journal of Psychiatry*, **112,** 9.

SEIDEN, R. H. (1966). Campus tragedy: a study of student suicide. *Journal of Abnormal and Social Psychology*, **71,** 389.

SELIGMAN, M. E. P. (1973). *Helplessness*. San Francisco: Freeman.

SEWELL, W. H. & MUSSEN, P. H. (1952). The effects of feeding, weaning, and scheduling procedures on childhood adjustment and formation of oral symptoms. *Child Development*, **23,** 185.

SHOBEN, E. J. (1949). The assessment of parental attitudes in relation to child adjustment. *Genetic Psychology Monographs*, **39,** 101.

SILBER, E., HAMBURG, D. A., COELHO, G. V., MURPHEY, E. B., ROSENBURG, M. & PERLIN, L. I. (1961). Adaptive behaviour in competent adolescents. *Archives of General Psychiatry*, **5,** 354.

SILBERER, H. (1912). On symbol formation. In *Organisation and pathology of Thought*, edited by D. Rapaport. New York: Columbia University Press, 1951.

SILLITOE, A. (1959). *The Loneliness of the Long Distance Runner*. London: Allen & Co.

STANTON, A. & SCHWARTZ, M. (1954). *The Mental Hospital*. New York: Basic Books.

STEVENSON, I. (1957). Is the human personality more plastic in infancy and childhood? *American Journal of Psychiatry*, **114,** 2, 152.

SWANK, R. L. & MARCHAND, W. E. (1946). Combat neuroses: development of combat exhaustion. *Archives of Neurology and Psychiatry*, **55,** 236.

SYMONDS, P. M. (1939). *Psychology of Parent-Child Relationships*. New York: Appleton-Century-Crofts.

TAIT, A. C., HARPER, J. & MCCLATCHEY, W. T. (1957). Initial psychiatric illness in involutional women. *Journal of Mental Science*, **103,** 132.

TERMAN, L. M. & MILES, C. C. (1936). *Sex and Personality*. New York: McGraw-Hill.

TIZARD, B. (1962). The application of Luria's techniques to the study of normal school children. *Journal of Child Psychology and Psychiatry*, **3,** 175.

TORRANCE, E. P. (1963). *Education and the Creative Potential*. Minneapolis: University of Minneapolis Press.

VERPLANCK, W. S. (1955). The control of the content of conversation: Reinforcement of statements of opinion. *Journal of Abnormal and Social Psychology*, **51,** 668.

& WAPNER, S. (1954). *Personality through Perception*. New York: Harper.

WATSON, J. B. & RAYNER, R. (1920). Conditioned emotional reactions. *Journal of Experimental Psychology*, **3,** 1.

WEINER, H., THALER, M., REISER, M. F. & MIRSKY, I. A. (1957). Aetiology of the duodenal ulcer: 1) Relation of specific psychological characteristics to rate of gastric secretion. *Psychosomatic Medicine*, **19,** 1.

WERNER, H. (1948). *Comparative Psychology of Mental Development*. New York: Follet.

WERTHEIMER, M. (1945). *Productive Thinking*. New York: Harper.

WEXLER, D., MENDELSON, J., LEIDERMAN, P. H. & SOLOMON, P. (1957). Sensory deprivation. *American Journal of Psychiatry*, **114,** 4, 357.

WITKIN, H. A., LEWIS, H. B., HERTZMAN, M., MACKOVER, K., MEISSNER, P. B. & WARNER, S. (1954). *Personality through Perception*. New York: Harper.

WITTREICH, W. J. (1959). Visual perception and personality. *Scientific American*, **200,** 4, 56.

WOLF, S. & WOLFF, H. H. (1967). *Human Gastric Function*. London: Oxford University Press.

WOODY, E. & CLARIDGE, G. (1977). Psychoticism and thinking. *British Journal of Social Clinical Psychology*, **16,** 241.

WOOTTON, B. (1959). *Social Science and Social Pathology*. London: Allen & Unwin.

ZIMBARDO, P. G. (1969). The human choice: individuation, reason and order versus deindividuation, impulse and chaos. In *Nebraska Symposium on Motivation*, edited by W. J. Arnold & D. Levine. Lincoln: University of Nebraska Press.

The Work of the Mental Nurse. A survey organized by a joint committee of the Manchester Regional Hospital Board and the University of Manchester: Manchester University Press, 1955.

Report of the Expert Committee on Psychiatric Nursing. *World Health Organization Technical Report Series*, 1957.

Two Year Old Goes to Hospital. A scientific film by James Robertson, research worker, Tavistock Clinic, London. (*See* ROBERTSON, J. (1953). Some responses of young children to loss of maternal care. *Nursing Times*, 18th April.)

Index

CHURCHILL LIVINGSTONE NURSING TEXTS

Nutrition and Dietetics for Nurses
Sixth edition
Mary E. Beck

Practical Therapeutics for Nursing and Related Professions
Third edition
James A. Boyle
Revised by David A. Henry and William R. Greig

Practical Notes on Nursing Procedures
Seventh edition
J. D. Britten

Bacteriology and Immunity for Nurses
Fifth edition
Ronald Hare and E. Mary Cooke

Drugs and Pharmacology for Nurses
Seventh edition
S. J. Hopkins

Essentials of Paediatrics for Nurses
Fifth edition
I. Kessel

A Nurse's Guide to Anaesthetics, Resuscitation and Intensive Care
Sixth edition
Walter Norris and *D. Campbell*

Anatomy and Physiology Applied to Nursing
Fifth edition
Janet T. E. Riddle

Principles of Nursing
Second edition
Nancy Roper

Foundations of Nursing and First Aid
Fifth edition
Janet S. Ross and *Kathleen J. W. Wilson*

Sociology and Nursing
First edition
James P. Smith

Pharmacology for Nurses
Seventh edition
J. R. Trounce